Understanding And Utilizing The Homoeopathic Materia Medica

Dr. Mir Zahed

Honorary Lecturer: Homoeopathic Academy of Niagara, Canada

Lecturer: Chiniot Homoeopathic Medical College, Chiniot, Pakistan

Founder, General Secretary: Organon Homoeopathic Medical Assocciation, Pakistan

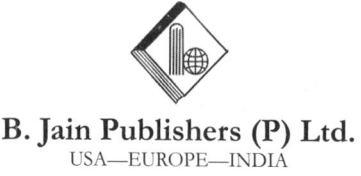

B. Jain Publishers (P) Ltd.
USA—EUROPE—INDIA

Understanding And Utilizing The Homoeopathic Materia Medica

Fifth Edition: 2013
2nd Impression: 2020

All rights reserved. No part of this book may be reproduced, stored in a retrieval system or transmitted, in any form or by any means, mechanical, photocopying, recording or otherwise, without any prior written permission of the publisher.
© with the author

Published by Kuldeep Jain for
B. JAIN PUBLISHERS (P) LTD.
1921/10, Chuna Mandi, Paharganj, New Delhi 110 055 (INDIA)
Tel.: +91-11-4567 1000 • Fax: +91-11-4567 1010
Email: info@bjain.com • Website: **www.bjain.com**
Printed in India by
J.J. Offset Printers

ISBN: 978-81-319-3035-9

Dedicated
To
Hahnemann
and
His Faithful Followers

Of whom one was my late teacher Mian Asghar Javed (Faisalabad). He was the first to teach me the principle of TOTALITY and turn me to righ path in HOMOEOPATHY.

"When we have to do with an art whose end is the saving of human life, any neglect to make ourselves thoroughly master of it becomes a crime."

Hahnemann
(Kent's Lesser Writings, P. 492)

Gratitude

Dr. Kathy Desjardins, founder and director of HOMOEOPATHIC ACADEMY OF NIAGARA, CANADA deserves my thanks twice. Firstly, because her keen interest in my lectures on Homoeopathic Materia Medica and other Homoeopathic works moulded me to compose these lectures for the students of her academy. Secondly, because she gladly and friendly offered to proofread this book in order to make it worth reading and useful for all students, beginners and those fond of HOMOEOPATHY.

I am also greatly thankful to respectable Dr. Ahmad Hassan Chaudhery (Sargodha, Pakistan) for having gone through the typescript word by word and making a number of corrections and suggestions. His corrections enhanced not only utility of the book but also my writing ability. I salute him for his sincere, affectionate and knowledgeable guidance with encouragement.

Respected Dr. Niel Madhavan, (Bomby, India) too, deserves my gratitude for studying the script keenly and making corrections, changes and additions to improve the quality and efficacy of the book.

And lastly I thank Dr. Kathy Thomas (Newzealand) for suggesting me to add a chapter on "Dose" which, I think, was quite necessary for beginners particularly those who are studying and practicing Kentian teachings.

Introductory

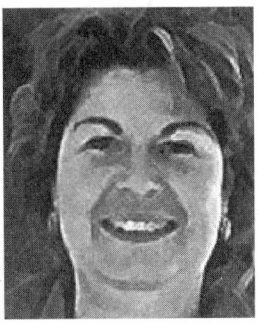

Kathy Desjardins (Canada)

Dr. Mir and I began corresponding some time ago in relation to his desire to teach at the Homoeopathic Academy of Niagara, in Canada. He delivered here (via internet and phone) some useful lectures and then our planned topic was "How to study Materia Medica. When he started writing on this topic it became a book.

Upon reading this work I was very impressed with the information that Dr. Mir had written. For beginning students of Homoeopathy, as we know, there are very few good books that one can find to start on his studies. Either the books are for general purposes, like first aid, or they are too in depth of new studies of this profession.

Dr. Mir's "UNDERSTANDING & UTILIZING The Homoeopathic Materia Medica" is an excellent book for beginning students of Homoeopathic Medicine. As a teacher of Homoeopathic Medicine I find the information that Dr. Mir has presented here an excellent starting point for my students. The messages are clear, concise and give a wonderful introduction into the complex studies of Homoeopathic Medicine.

I highly recommend that all students who have started on their journey of Homoeopathic Medicine should read this book. In addition I suggest that all Homoeopathic Schools should recommend this book on the required reading list for year one.

It is with great honor, thanks and appreciation that I write these words for Dr. Mir.

Yours truly,
Kathy Desjardins
Director
Homoeopathic Academy of Niagara (Canada)

Foreword

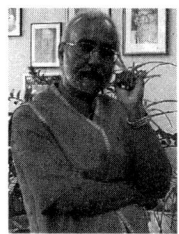

Dr. Mohinder Singh Jus (SHI Switzerland)

Materia Medica cannot and should not be memorized but understood. This is the main theme so excellently discussed in this book. It is written in the tradition of Dr. Kent who taught us to understand the homoeopathic remedies as personalities. Being myself a Kentian Homoeopath and teacher, I read this book with great joy and was pleased to write the foreword.

The author explains his method to read and understand materia medica and includes view points of renowned homoeopaths. He illustrates this subject with very valuable examples. He emphasizes about the importance of understanding all aspects of a remedy such as source of the remedy, characteristic symptoms, general and particular symptoms, duration of action and comparison with other remedies. Interestingly he elaborates the importance of knowing the source of a drug, as to why it affects particularly on specific systems or organs and how it reflects certain similarity to another drug. He recommends that the remedies should be studied under various groups e.g. "cold remedies; hot remedies". This helps the homoeopath to select the correct remedy.

For a beginner, it is always difficult to grasp the method of evaluation of symptoms. Dr. Zahed skilfully emphasizes the importance of gradation of symptoms in the Kentian way that is mental symptoms, generals and locals. He underlines the significance of modalities in the selection of a remedy. He has thoroughly discussed the subject of drug relationship. This is a much disputed subject. Some of the modern homoeopaths even do not consider it of any importance. They find the mention of complementary, follow-up remedies, inimicals or antidotes as irrelevant. I personally think that it is a shame to ignore the centuries old experience of innumerable renowned and dedicated homoeopaths who witnessed these effects in their busy clinics. It is a great compliment to Dr. Zahed for having laid emphasis on such a subject which is vast and very useful. To select the right remedy alone is not enough. It is its comprehensive use and follow-up of the case which is challenging. In my experience, in order to accomplish a cure, it is imperative to take into account the drug relationships. They are like a compass to the treating homoeopath.

After having extensively discussed the drug relationships, the author goes into another very important subject: the potencies. He has given very interesting and valuable viewpoints of various homoeopaths. This should be very helpful in determining the correct potency as to the gravity of the case and personal sensitivity of the patient.

All in all this work from Dr. Zahed will go a long way to help all the beginners and advance students of homoeopathy. With its easily comprehensible language and text, this book is a big service to the homoeopathic profession. I wish Dr. Zahed all the best and congratulate him for his achievement.

Dr. Mohinder Singh Jus, DMS (Cal)

Director: SHI Homoeopathic College and Clinic
Editor: Similia, Quarterly Homoeopathic Journal
Lecturer: SHI Homoeopathic College and in various foreign countries
Author: Journey of a Disease, A Comprehensive Study of Miasms, Children Types, Practical Materia Medica etc.

Preface

Many of the articles which make up this book were originally prepared and delivered (via internet) as lectures to the students of Homoeopathic Academy of Niagara, CANADA. Dr. Kathy Desjardins, founder and director of the academy and many of my students and friends expressed their belief that publishing of these lectures in book form will serve a useful purpose. So now this work (revised and expanded) is presented to all lovers of homoeopathy. I hope students and beginners of Homoeopathy will surely gain something useful from this book.

It is not uncommon that many people, inspired by miracles of Homoeopathy, are eagerly inclined to study and practice Homoeopathic Materia Medica. But not being familiar with Homeopathic philosophy they cannot comprehend and grasp it. So in this work I have tried to elucidate the philosophical basis and importance of constituents of the Homoeopathic Materia Medica. The object is twofold. Firstly, to enable the reader to comprehend Materia Medica and to pick out the essential features of every remedy which depict its comprehensible and practicable picture. Secondly, to make the reader know that Materia Medica can neither be understood nor utilized without Philosophy.

In this work I have no claim of presenting my original thoughts. However I have collected material on the subject scattered in a large number of authentic books on Homoeopathic Philosophy and Materia Medica. In this I tried to generate maximum understanding of the subject in minimun text. Our most classical literature is too heavy to understand for a beginner. I tried to explain the basic concepts in an easy and comprehensible way. So I hope the book will be a useful addition to the literature of Homoeopathy—the only true healing system. According to my present knowledge I tried my best to cover most aspects of the subject. Yet I warmly welcome suggestions from Homoeopathic fraternity to make it more useful to our posterity.

Mir Zahed
Chiniot
21-02-2008

Publisher's Note

Studying Materia Medica and remembering it is a herculean task, that is why Dr Kent suggested use of repertory. But even to use a repertory one has to be well versed with Materia Medica as its rightly said "you will search only what you know". There are different ways of studying Materia Medica but the finest way is going back to classical works and understanding remedies through stalwart's eyes. This is exactly what Dr Mir has done, that is, elaborated a way to study Materia Medica by use of classical books. He has painstakingly picked all the basic books and explained the best way to read and use each one of them and thus apply that into practice. He has made reading Materia Medica an interesting affair. This book shall serve as a teaching tool for all the aspirants who wish to learn Materia Medica through right way. This book shall be enlisted as one of the reference works and teaching tool for the said subject.

Kuldeep Jain
CEO, B. Jain Publishers

Contents

Introductory	*ix*
Foreword	*xi*
Preface	*xiii*
1. **Materia Medica to Memorize or to Understand!**	1
2. **Source and Kingdom**	5
3. **Relation to Heat and Cold**	15
4. **Acute or Chronic Remedy**	17
5. **Remedy's Specific Action and Relation to Specific Organs of the Body**	21
6. **Symptoms**	25
General Symptoms	27
Importance of General Symptoms	27
Types of General Symptoms	30
(a) Mental/Emotional Symptoms	30
(b) Physical General Symptoms	33
(c) Food Symptoms	34
(d) Sex Symptoms	36
(e) Sleep Symptoms	36
(f) Chief Complaint	37
(g) Pathological General Symptoms (Pathological Predispositions or Tendencies)	37
Particular Symptoms	40
Pathological Symptoms	42

Common and Uncommon Symptoms	50
Concomitant Symptoms	55
Keynote Symptoms	56
Subjective and Objective Symptoms	59
7. Modalities	**61**
Important Factors of Modalities	66
8. Causations	**69**
9. Duration of Action	**75**
10. Relationship of Remedies	**77**
Complementary Remedies	77
Remedies That Follow Well	78
Inimical Remedies	79
Antidote Remedies	80
11. Comparison with Resemblinng Remedies	**85**
12. Study of Cured Cases	**87**
13. The Appropriate Potency	**89**
Start and Gradual Development of The Potency System	91
Scales of Homoeopathic Potencies	94
Decimal Scale	94
Centesimal Scale	94
Fifty-Millesimal Scale	94
Necessity and Advantage of Maximum Range of Potencies	96
Required Range of Potencies as Suggested by Experts	98
General Guidelines For Different Degrees of Potencies	99

High Potencies	99
Medium Potencies	101
Low Potencies	104
Conclusion	107
14. Dose (Administration of Medicine)	**115**
15. Study of Repertory	**135**
16. Literature on Homoeopathic Materia Medica	**137**
Elementary Stage	138
Middle Stage	138
Advance Stage	139
17. Study Plan	**141**
Level 1	142
Level 2	143
Level 3	144
18. Sample Study	**145**
Leaders in Homoeopathic Therapeutics	**145**
By: E.B. Nash	*145*
Nux Vomica	150
Homoeopathic Drug Pictures	**158**
By: M.L. Tyler	*158*
Argentum Nitricum	161
Lectures on Materia Medica & Comparative Study on Kent's Matria Medica	**169**
By: J.T. Kent & A.Gaskin	*169*
Carbo Vegetabilis (J.T. Kent)	177
Carbo Vegetabilis (A. Gaskin)	201

Lectures on Clinical Materia Medica in Family Order	**208**
By: E.A. Farrington M.D.	208
Sepia (I)	221
Key Notes of Leading Remedies	**236**
By: H.C. Allen	236
Pulsatilla	238
Keynotes of the Homoeopathic Materia Medica	**241**
By: Dr. Adolph Von Lippe	241
Natrum Muriaticum	242
The Genius of Homoeopathic Remedies	**247**
By: Dr. S.M. Gunavante	247
Sulphur	248
Pocket Manual of the Homoeopathic Materia Medica	**254**
By: William Boericke, M.D.	254
Lycopodium Clavatum (Club Moss)	257
A Study on Materia Medica	**264**
By: N.M. Choudhuri	264
Aloe Socotrina	266
Materia Medica of Homoeopathic Medicines	**271**
By: S.R. Phatak	271
China Officinalis	273
Bibliography	**278**
Reviews	**280**
Dr. Ahmad Hassan Choudhery, Sargodha, Pakistan	280
Dr. Manish Bhatia, Jaipur, India	280

Dr. Kathy Thomas, Newzealand 281
Dr. Navneet Bidani, New Delhi, India 282
Dr. Niel Madhavan, Mumbai, India 283

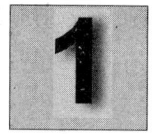

MATERIA MEDICA: TO MEMORIZE OR TO UNDERSTAND!

Homoeopathic practice depends on three things
  (1) Homoeopathic Philosophy
  (2) Homoeopathic Materia Medica
  (3) Homoeopathic Repertory

Homoeopathic Philosophy is based on the Organon which is difficult to understand for some reasons. However when it is keenly studied we can understand and practice it successfully.

Repertory work is also a matter of reading and exercising. When we have understood the purpose and structure of a Repertory, by its constant study and use we can become well acquainted with it.

But the actual problem comes with Materia Medica. What is Materia Medica? It is a record of the effects of medicinal substances on healthy human beings that are called symptoms. One medicinal substance has been proven to produce hundreds and some times thousands of symptoms that apparently have no connection to each other. The more one goes into the details of these thousands of incoherent symptoms the more one gets confused in understanding them or retaining them in the mind. Thus Homoeopathic Materia Medica seems a dry study and it is impossible to absorb it fully. Even if Hahnemann's "Materia Medica Pura" is put into the hands of a beginner, he will be frightened away from the study of Homoeopathic Materia Medica and will abandon Homoeopathy.

We can say that Philosophy and Repertory always guide us in the practice, whereas we have always to chase Materia Medica. If someone, without understanding this dilemma and finding its solution, tries to read through all of the Materia Medica he exerts unnecessary mental labour; he may waste his five or ten precious years, and still not be able to recognize the precise remedy from the Materia Medica for the patient in hand. Firstly because it is very hard to read all of the Materia Medicas and secondly mere reading is not sufficient. That's why, our experts say, Materia Medica should not be memorized but understood. J.T. Kent says in the preface to his Lectures on Materia Medica,

"Materia Medica can be learned by careful study and by using it. It can be understood but not memorized. All who would try to memorize the Materia Medica must ignominiously fail."

(J.T. Kent, Lectures on Materia Medica P. 12)

Now the question rises as to how we can understand and comprehend it enough to take it into practice. In this regard we find different suggestions and viewpoints in our literature. Hahnemann directs us to the strange, rare and uncommon symptoms. J.T. Kent and Lippe forcefully emphasize on general symptoms. Farrington builds his "Clinical Materia Medica" in family order and describes number of properties and symptoms of drugs accordingly. Rajan Sankaran finds the qualities and properties of remedies from their source and kingdom. Materia Medicas by E.B. Nash, J.T.Kent, M.L. Tyler and George Vithoulkas have been designed in descriptive form so that a coherent picture of the remedy may come before the reader to recognize the remedies and retain that information. But any of these methods alone does not meet needs of a homoeopath. One does not fit all cases. For a successful practice we need to know a remedy from many aspects.

We can understand a remedy well if we ponder over every aspect of it that can be helpful for us in gaining the knowledge of its qualities and properties. According to my knowledge and experience, if we are aware of the following aspects of Materia Medica we may apply it properly:

- Source and kingdom
- Relation to heat and cold
- Acute or chronic nature of remedy
- Relation to specific organs and specific action of remedy
- Symptoms (gradation and classification)
- Modalities
- Causations
- Duration of action
- Relationship of remedies
- Comparison with resembling remedies
- Study of cured cases
- The appropriate potency
- Dose (administration of medicine)

2

SOURCE AND KINGDOM

First of all, after the name, we should know what are source, origin and kingdom of a remedy. (Vegetable, Mineral or Animal). Many times the source and origin of a remedy provide us with a very useful knowledge of its qualities and properties. P.Sankaran in his booklet "The Study of Materia Medica" has given very interesting information of many remedies related to their source and origin. To quote him,

"Such aspects like the morphology, habitat, physical and chemical properties, family relationships, group tendencies, the identity of substances, the source and origin with particular reference to the nature and behavior of the original substance (mineral, plant and animal). Traditional uses, physiological and toxic effects, medicinal and non-medicinal uses etc, should be considered and analyzed. Every piece of information that may enhance our understanding of the drugs should be collected and collated".

(P.Sankaran, The Study of Materia Medica, P. 7)

"Habitat has a great part in such moulding. Members of the animal and vegetable kingdom acquire certain properties by virtue of the soil and climate wherein they flourish, the quantity and quality of nourishment, water and sunlight they receive, etc. In this respect, they may be compared to human beings whose characteristics, habits and reactions are often moulded by the circumstances and environment of their life. Animals and even plants develop special methods of sustenance and self-protection suitable to the areas wherein they reside. One would almost think them to be human and that their behavior is as much the result of intelligence as of instinct. All these inherited and acquired virtues and defects go to make up the individuality of the substances, which is reflected in their actions and reactions. It is also considered by some that substances available on the spot are usually found most suitable to diseases arising in that area, as for example, Arnica Montana found in mountainous regions is a unique remedy both for the exertion and after-effects of mountain climbing as also for the injuries sustained by climbers from falls. Aconite grows in dry soil and its symptoms are worse in dry weather. The idea is that the influences that go to produce the diseases peculiar to the place also go to mould the drugs peculiar to the place, which may prove useful for such types of diseases.

"The chemical composition of substances often explains their action, e.g. the action of Spongia resembles that of Iodum closely, the latter being a constituent of the former substance. Both are better by eating. Ledermann says that the iodine component of Spongia can account for its effects on swellings of the testicle and epididymis. Lycopodium contains sulphur and hence much of its similarity to Sulphur, the close relationship of Pulsatilla and Kali sulph, arises from the fact that Pulsatilla contains potassium sulphate. Lycopodium contains both Silica and Aluminium and has symptoms of both the drugs such as diffidence, constipation with soft but difficult stool etc., Antimonium crudum contains sulphur and has similar aversion to and aggravation from bath and heat. Allium cepa also contains sulphur and has similar acrid discharge. Both Graphites and Petroleum contain carbon and have symptoms like Carbo vegetabilis. Graphites contains in addition 3% of iron and has several symptoms of Ferrum in its pathogenesis. Kreosote also contains carbon and has black, offensive, burning discharges. Nux vomica contains copper and has all the spasms and cramps of Cuprum. Both Nux vom. and Ignatia contain strychnine and produce similar convulsions. Belladonna contains Magnesium phosphate, and has spasms and pains."

(P.Sankaran, The Study of Materia Medica, PP. 9-11)

Farrington says,

"A study of the vegetable kingdom involves to some extent a study of the mineral kingdom, because many of the medicinal properties of vegetable remedies owe their existence to substances derived from the minerals in the soil in which they grow. The principal effectes of some of the grasses are the result of the large quantity of Silica they contain. Ninety-nine one-hundreds of the effects of Laurocerasus come from its Hydrocyanic or Prussic acid, which is commonly classed with the inorganic compounds. The same may be said of Amygdala persica. Now these substances derived from the mineral kingdom and contained in the vegetable kingdom, become more active in their new environment; that is to say, a given chemical substance, if made synthetically in the laborotary, would possess less marked medicinal virtues than if it were obtained from a plant."

(Farrington, Clinical Materia Medica, PP. 177-78)

Farrinton has connected properties and symtopms of many medicines to their chemical components. Here are some examples,

"Graphites is an impure carbon which contains traces of Iron. It combines the offensive secretions, flatulency and skin symptoms of the carbons, with anemia".

(Farrington, Clinical Materia Medica, P. 154)

(Natrum Carb) "At other times, the patient suffers from diarrhea. The stool is papescent or watery, with violent urging. This characteristic of the soda salts, you will find to be quite general. You find it also in Natrium Sulph. It seems to be due to the purgative effect of the soda itself. Wine in such cases, as this causes faintness and vertigo, not agreeing with the patient at all."

(Farrington, Clinical Materia Medica, P. 844)

(Kaki Carb) "There is an aggravation of all the symptoms from three to five o' clock in the morning. This hour of aggravation belongs to all the potash salts."

(Farrington, Clinical Materia Medica, P. 908)

P.Sankaran goes on exploring the therapeutic points of remedies known by their source and origin and quotes some authorities like Hubbard, Grimmer and Stonham etc. He writes with their references as,

"That marvelous teacher Hubbard writes, "To simplify Materia Medica one must ponder on the elements of which all other substances and man is made, one must analyze plants based on their component parts at least the predominant ones and feel one's way into the relationship of remedies. Who is not helped by knowing that Lachesis contains much sulphur? Or Lycopodium a lot of alumina? Or Bell. some magnesium phosphoricum and Nux vomica a share of copper?" Lapis albus is nothing but Calcium silico-fluoride and so covers tumours of bones. Pulsatilla contains Iron and both Pulsatilla and Ferrum have many common symptoms and are indicated in anaemic patients who are better by slow motion. Borax being Sodium Biborate belongs to the Natrum family and has similar aggravation from noise. Causticum, being a potassium compound has the weakness of the Kali group, extending to paralysis. Grimmer says Merc.sol. contains traces of Nitric acid; both are aggravated at night and are prominently anti-syphilitic. Analyzing the action of salts Stonham says, "The analysis showed that in all cases the basic element predominates in its salt. The salt is more than the sum of the qualities of the elements that compose it. We may perhaps infer that the chlorides work in the direction of the arterial system, the bromides of the sexual organs, the iodides of the lymphatics and glands and the phosphates skeletal and nervous systems, while the sulphates have a more general influence on the system generally. It may be that when we have a more certain knowledge of the correlation between the physiological action of drugs and their chemical structure we shall be able to make a better prediction of the therapeutic value of their combinations".

The family and group tendencies are also prominent, such as the sadness of the Natrums, the weakness of the Kalis, the neuralgic pains of the Magnesium family, the sluggishness of the Carbons, the glandular affections of the Halogens, the prostration of the Acids and so on".

(P.Sankaran, The Study of Materia Medica, P. 11)

Farrington designed his materia medica in family order and mentioned many common properties and symptoms of different families of medicines; here are some examples,

(Absinthium) "In the delirium the patient is obliged to walk about. You will note this symptom running through all the remedies of the order. Chamommilla and Cina have relief from moving about; Artemisia has desire to move about; and here under Absinthium the patient walks about in distress, seeing all sorts of visions"

(Farrington, Clinical Materia Medica, P. 276)

"(Cucurbitaceae) Of the medicinal substances obtained from this order we may say that they all act prominently on the alimentary tract. They seem to have in common a cathartic action. They probably act paralyzingly on the vaso-motor nerves of the abdomen. They produce griping pains, gushing watery diarrhoea. This last symptom is most prominent under Elaterium".

(Farrington, Clinical Materia Medica, P. 327)

Let us read a little more from P. Sankaran's "The Study of Materia Medica" and see how source and origin of remedies provide us with their useful therapeutic points,

"By the identity of substances is meant the knowledge what they actually are. Sometimes the Homoeopathic Materia Medica is studied without a proper knowledge of the identity of the substances studied. One who has seen the jelly-like content of the Aloe leaves will remember the identical nature of the discharges produced and removed by the drug; one who has eaten the root-tubers of the Arum plant (Yam) especially the raw or partly cooked state, will not forget the terrible rawness accompanied by great itching that it produces in the throat. Mercury on being dropped scatters itself in a restless manner reminding us of the restless patient requiring Mercurius solubilis. Can we not understand the lachrymation and coryza of Allium cepa when we know it is the onion that has made cooks lachrymose? Similarly we can appreciate the foetid discharges of Asafoetida; the pride under Platinum, the most expensive and therefore a proud metal; the aggravation from petrol fumes and car-sickness of Petroleum; the burning redness and pungency of Capsicum, the cayenne pepper etc."

(P.Sankaran, The Study of Materia Medica, PP. 12-13)

"Knowledge of the source and origin of substances helps much. Sulphur comes from burning lava of the volcanoes and produces much burning. Amphisboena is prepared from the jawbone of the lizard and acts markedly on the jaw. For substances of animal origin, quite often the behaviour and habits of the animals give a clue to their action and uses. It is said that the Lachesis snake coils itself always from left to right, in which direction the symptoms of the drug also travel".

We know the snake does not make its own burrow; it always occupies a hole made by some other animal, so how much jealousy and malice we see in Lachesis.

"One who has read about the habits of the Tarentula spider will easily comprehend the cunningness and quickness of the spider reflected in its symptomatology. Persons bitten become more or less insane every spring and then on hearing the least musical sound, start dancing wildly. Though the music thus aggravates their condition at first, later they feel greatly relieved after they continuously dance for three or four days and become thoroughly exhausted. This is why, in Homoeopathic Repertories, this drug is given under the rubrics "Agg. From music" and "Amel. from music and dancing".

The nature of the drug is also very useful. Drosera is an insectivorous plant. Whenever a fly sits on the leaf, the leaf slowly closes, imprisons the fly and secretes a juice that is able to digest the fly. It is also able, similarly, to dissolve bones and glands as in tuberculosis. Further, sheep eating Drosera leaves develop a nocturnal cough and die. Dros. is a well-known remedy for cough at night and for tubercular glands. The plant Rhus-tox is said to be most poisonous in rainy weather and symptoms of that drug are worse in that weather. Pulsatilla, also known as the windflower, is a remedy for women who are reputedly changeable like the wind. Natrum mur. being salt produces a lot of thirst. Potassium has a toxic effect on the heart and Kali carb. presents many heart symptoms. Apis is derived from the honeybee. The queen bee is a most jealous creature, so jealous that after cohabitation with a male bee it kills the drone because it cannot tolerate the idea of the drone having relationship with some other female bee, with the results that it is itself widowed. So Apis is a remedy for the effects of jealousy and for widows.

The traditional and other uses of the drugs also give much information. Bellis Perennis (Daisy) is used as a remedy for injuries. Even after being trampled upon, the flowers come up smiling. Aloe has been traditionally used for inducing abortion because it is able to bring out everything involuntarily, including the stool and the rectum. Bufo had been made use of to produce impotence by women who found their husbands sexually overactive. Stramonium has been given to produce insanity, Opium has been used to produce constipation and sense of well being and when these symptoms are found in the sick, it is able to cure. Coffee is taken to produce insomnia, e.g. by students preparing for examination, and it is our well known remedy for insomnia, Nux moschata is used by village women to keep children quiet and drowsy while they go away for work. Cannabis indica is taken by addicts to experience glorious delusions and fantasies. Carbo veg. is used in modern medicine for flatulence since it has the capacity to absorb 40 times its volume of gas. Merc. Sol. is used in thermometers and barometers to indicate the changes of temperature and weather; the Merc.sol. patients also react as quickly to such changes. Belladonna (Bella=beautiful, Donna=lady) was being used by women to produce brightness of the eyes and red cheeks so that they may look attractive. It produces all these symptoms in the individual along with hot head and cold extremities. Curare the famous arrow poison is used to catch animals alive since it paralyses the hind legs of running animals."

(P. Sankaran, The Study of Materia Medica, PP. 13-16)

In this way we get a very useful knowledge of the effects of medicinal substances through their source and kingdom. But it does not mean that source or kingdom provides us the complete knowledge of symptoms, properties and qualities of remedies. Symptoms, properties and qualities of medicinal substances can be fully known only by their provings on healthy human beings according to the instructions of Master Hahnemann.

However the knowledge derived from source and kingdom is useful to a good extent in understanding and applying our Materia Medica.

In the selection of potency and mode of its repetition kingdom also plays an important role. Most acute remedies belong to vegetable kingdom such as Aconit, Arnica, Chamomilla, and Gelsemium etc. But this is not always the rule because some plant remedies are deep/long acting such as Carbo veg, Lycopodium and Thuja etc.

Animal poisons and nosodes, such as Lachesis, Naja and Medorrhinum, are capable of producing heavy pathological changes on physical level and thus require more caution in potency selection and repetition. Vithoulkas says,

"Another mistaken idea is that no harm can be done if a beginning prescriber restricts potencies to below 30. As previously mentioned, any potency can have profound actions depending upon the similarity of the medicine to the patient. If the remedy is the similimum, even a crude dose or a very low potency can have profound effect; indeed, if it is originally a poisonous substance and it closely matches the resonant frequency of an oversensitive patient, a lower potency can produce a severe and dangerous aggravation.

There are a few remedies which one should be cautious about giving high potencies. Medicines such as Lachesis, Aurum, and deep-acting nosodes (especially Medorrhinum) have strong tendencies toward physical pathology. For this reason, they should usually be restricted to lower potencies (30 or 200) unless the individual case is demonstrated to be quite free of physical pathology".

(G. Vithoulkas, The Science of Homoeopathy, PP.216-17)

Mineral remedies are the most deeply and long acting and thus need circumspection and caution in repetition and choice of potency, particularly those that cause heavy tissue changes such as Arsenic or Mercurius etc.

Remedies like Silicea, Phosphorus and Sulphur which tear off the tissues and throw unnecessary matters out of the body must be used with great caution and circumspection in the last stages of tuberculosis, chronic severe arthritis and valvular disease---- diseases with severe tissue changes. Kent warns us against using high potencies of these remedies in such conditions,

"Phosphorus is a dangerous medicine to give very high in some cases of phthisis, in the last stages of phthisis. In this case they should have received Phosphorus when they were yet curable. In these cases Phosphorus 30th may sometimes be used with safety and it will act as a test in doubtful cases to see whether reaction can be brought about. In such cases where reaction can be brought about the administration later of a still higher potency may be found useful, but in the beginning with Phosphorus in phthisical cases far advanced it is better not to go higher than the 30th or 200th. Phosphorus very low will act as a poison in really Phosphorus cases and the only safety some patients have had who have received Phosphorus so very low was due to the fact that the Phosphorus was not similar enough to either kill or cure".

(J.T. Kent, Lectures on Materia Medica, P. 834)

If there is a deposit of tubercle in the lungs, Silica establishes an inflammation and throws it out, and if the whole lung be tubercular a general suppurative pneumonia will be the result; hence, the danger of giving such remedies and the danger of repeating them in advanced stage of phthisis. Not only Silica but many other remedies have the power to suppurate out deposits, the result of poor nutrition".

(J.T. Kent, Lectures on Materia Medica, P. 927)

"Sulphur is, perhaps, the better remedy to prevent suppuration when there are not typhoid symptoms, but be careful how you give Sulphur if tuberculosis has been developed by pneumonia. To do so is almost like giving a person running down hill another push. It will only hasten the end".

(Farrington, Clinical Materia Medica, P. 44)

It is necessary to clear here that the above noted precautions apply particularly to centesimal potencies and the dosage based on the 4th and 5th Organon upon which Kent based his practice. In the 6th Organon Hahnemann converted to Fifty Millesimal (LM) potencies which proved to be greatly useful in all such cases of advanced pathology. The Homoeopathic Physician will be spared many a consciousness pangs if he uses the advanced dosing methodologies explained in the 6th Organon. We shall discuss this issue in detail in the chapter "Dose" (Administration of Medicine).

3

RELATION TO HEAT AND COLD

Connection and relation of a remedy or a patient to thermal conditions on the whole is very important and should always be considered essentially. Firstly, because being affected either by Heat or by Cold, on the whole, is a physical general symptom and no cure can be effected or expected if Physical General Symptoms are opposite or Contra-indicating in the remedy chosen and the patient in hand. For example we have a patient with some important symptoms of Arsenic Alb. viz extreme restlessness with anxiety, fear of death and agg. at night but he feels better in cold and is aggravated by heat in general. Then in spite of these strong features of Arsenic, it will not be a curative remedy for him. Arsenic may palliate for some length of time (because of partial similarity) but will not cause a complete cure.

Secondly, the relation of a remedy or a patient to heat or cold in general facilitates the selection. If a patient is decidedly sensitive to and aggravated by heat, in general, then it is must to select a remedy for him from the group of Hot/Warm remedies. It means only this one symptom will put two third of all the Materia Medica aside, and if we combine one or two more general symptoms with it, there will be a very short list of remedies before us from all the Materia Medica. From that very short list we will find the required remedy in no time.

In this way all our Materia Medica (except very few remedies especially those small remedies that do not disturb the organism on physical general level and therefore have no relation to Heat and Cold) is divided into three parts:

- Cold Remedies
- Warm or Hot remedies
- Both (Ambivalent) Remedies

The patients who are aggravated by or sensitive to heat in general their remedy will be selected from the Hot/Warm group. In the same way for a cold patient remedy will always be selected from cold group; and for a patient sensitive to or aggravated by both heat and cold remedy will be selected from the remedies called both/ambivalent.

In this regard we should consult rubrics of Heat and Cold agg. in Generalities chapter of repertory books. Dr.Gibson Miller's list of Hot and Cold remedies given at the start of Kent's Repertory is also very helpful. We can also consult the chart of miasmatic and heat and cold remedies at the end of S.K. Banerjea's book "Miasmatic Diagnosis"

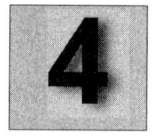

ACUTE OR CHRONIC REMEDY

Like Acute and Chronic Diseases some remedies in our Materia Medica are Acute, limited and superficial whereas some others are Chronic—very deep, long acting and extensive. Acute diseases and conditions are treated with acute remedies whereas Chronic Miasmatic diseases can be uprooted only with the help of chronic and deep acting remedies. For fast and violent conditions like Cholera or Sunstroke we shall definitely need quick and fast remedies like Veratrum Alb and Glonoine, whereas chronic miasmatic diseases and conditions due to Psora, Sycosis and Syphilis can only be cured with the help of deep anti-miasmatic remedies like Sulphur, Thuja and Mercurius. Obviously we shall need as deep and extensive remedies as the conditions we are facing. Neither superficial, limited and short acting remedies can cure chronic and deep diseases nor acute, superficial and transient diseases need deep anti-miasmatic remedies. We can say a true homoeopath neither tries hunting of lions with the help of a pellet-gun nor thinks of dropping a bomb to kill a lizard.

Thus in studying Materia Medica we should also keep this point in mind whether the remedy belongs merely to acute and superficial conditions or is capable of curing deep chronic miasmatic diseases. Even Kent, one of the most intelligent and skillful Homoeopaths, has to say that when he did not know that Asthma is a manifestation of sycosis he used to think it incurable. But when he came to know this fact he could cure patients of asthma by applying anti-sycotic remedies like Thuja, Medorrhinum and Natrum Sulp. etc.

But to recognize the symptoms of miasms in Materia Medica and to know which remedy belongs to which miasm, firstly we must be well acquainted with the detailed symptomatology of miasms. We cannot understand the relationship of any remedy with any miasm unless we know which miasm produces what kind of symptoms and conditions.

For this purpose, besides rubrics of miasms in the repertory books, one should carefully study S.K. Banerjea's "Miasmatic Diagnosis". It gives us detailed symptoms of four miasms (Psora, Sycosis, Syphilis and Tubercular) in a chematic and comparative way. At end a beautiful chart highlights relation of remedies to relative miasms. Another beautiful book is "The Journey of a Disease" by a contemporary senior homoeopath Dr. Mohinder Singh Jus (SHI Switzerland). It gives an insight into miasmatic diseases and complicated conditions that occur after their suppression. But don't forget to study "The Chronic Diseases" by Dr. Hahnemann. This is the only source book that gives us basic understanding of chronic miasms.

Granted that relationship between the remedy and the miasm is an important factor for selection of remedy, final decision would always be taken on the basis of symptoms. Moreover it is not obligatory to select a superficial and limited (acute) remedy for an acute condition, because if there are symptoms of a deep remedy in an acute illness we are bound to select it. Some remedies in our Materia Medica possess nature of both acute and chronic diseases such as Arsenic, Lachesis and Merc Sol etc. If there are symptoms of a deep miasmatic remedy in an acute illness those will definitely be cured by it being the remedy more powerful than the disease. However acute and superficial remedies cannot cure deep chronic miasmatic diseases. Hahnemann says in aphorism No.103

"In the same manner as has here been taught relative to the epidemic diseases, which are generally of an acute character, the miasmatic chronic maladies, which, as I have shown, always remain the same in their essential nature, especially the Psora, must be investigated, as to the whole sphere of their symptoms, in a much more minute manner than has ever been done before, for in them also one patient only exhibits a portion of their symptoms, a second, a third, and so on, present some other symptoms, which also are but a (dissevered, as it were) portion of the totality of the symptoms which constitute the entire extent of this malady, so that the whole array of the symptoms belonging to such a miasmatic, chronic disease, and especially to the psora, can only be ascertained from the observation of very many single patients affected with such a chronic disease, and without a complete survey and collective picture of these symptoms the medicines capable of curing the whole malady homeopathically (to wit, the antipsorics) cannot be discovered; and these medicines are, at the same time, the true remedies of the several patients suffering from such chronic affections".

(Hahnemann, Organon of Medicine, aphorism 103 PP. 185-86)

Thus we should always keep in mind that superficial remedies like Glonoin and Gelsemium etc. cannot cure chronic miasmatic headaches. Rather to cure them we need deep anti-miasmatic remedies like Nat-m or Silicia etc. Deep and powerful remedies like Argentum Nit, Mercurius or Phosphorus cure chronic miasmatic infections of eyes instead of Euphrasia. Most neophytes give Aconite to every patient on the keynote symptoms of fear of death. But if the fear of death is in a chronic miasmatic patient we will definitely need some anti-miasmatic remedy like Arsenic and Argent-Nit etc. Kent says,

"He, who sees not in Brights' disease the deep miasm at the back of it, sees not the whole disease, but only the finishing of a long course of symptoms which have been developing for years"

(J.T. Kent, Lesser Writings, P. 659)

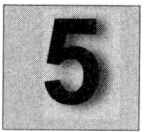

REMEDY'S SPECIFIC ACTION AND RELATION TO SPECIFIC ORGANS OF THE BODY

Every medicinal substance affects the man differently and causes changes in different organs in different ways. Thus the symptoms of every remedy are different. Therefore we should know and understand relation of every remedy to specific organs and its specific disease actions. No doubt symptoms, either in the remedy or in the patient, are prior to pathological and organic changes and Homoeopathic cure is based on the symptoms, and if symptoms were cured pathologies would be repaired themselves. But this does not mean that we should disregard the relation of the remedy to specific organs and its specific disease action. Certain authors like Kent, while emphasizing the importance of General Symptoms have so much disregarded the disease action and particular symptoms that the reader may lose absolutely their importance. But this is neither fully practicable nor Hahnemann has advised us to proceed in this fashion. He says in aphorism 18:

"The sum of all the symptoms and conditions in each individual case of disease must be the sole indication, the sole guide to direct us in the choice of the remedy".

(Hahnemann, Organon of Medicine P. 106)

It means disease is a totality of all symptoms and pathological conditions. Neither the name of the disease and pathological conditions can be the base of a true curative mode of treatment nor can merely general symptoms provide the complete picture of disease on which we choose the most appropriate Homoeopathic remedy. In the preface of "Leaders in Homoeopathic Therapeutics" Nash says,

"(I am offering this book) to try to discourage the disposition to quarrel over Symptomatology and Pathology. Neither can be ruled out, and it is foolish for our school to divide on such a bone of contention. Every symptom has its pathological significance, but we cannot always give it in words".

(Nash, Leaders in Homoeopathic Therapeutics P. 4)

In the early years of my practice I did make some mistakes on this point and had to face some failures. Since I corrected these mistakes percentage of my successful cases significantly increased. Symptoms are always considered important than pathologies. If a remedy appears to be indicated in a case according to other important symptoms but is not mentioned in the pathology, we would choose the remedy according to the patient and ignore the pathology. For instance a patient comes to us with the complaint of nasal polypus. He has also some important general and psychic symptoms which guide us to a particular medicine. But the medicine has not been recorded under polypus. The principle is that we will select that remedy and that will cure polypus too. If a patient has decidedly symptoms of a constitutional remedy but a remedy, like Lemna minor, merely on the basis of polypus is applied he will not be cured. Symptoms characrerize and are the basis of pathology; symptoms are always superior to pathology. However the best fitted Homoeopathic remedy is the one that covers both the symptoms and the pathology. We must keep every aspect in view to arrive at a curative medicine.

"It is not without reason that Hahnemann and Boennigheusen so zealously talked of Locations, Sensations, Modalities and Concomitants. All these must be taken care of by any medicine to be of any effect in curing the disease. The only exception, to my knowledge and experience are cases where we have to use a Nosode to open up the case by removing the blocks."

(Paragraph added by Dr. Niel Madhavan, Bombay, India)

C.M.Boger, in his "Synoptic Key to Materia Medica", has pointed out the centres of action of every remedy at the top, surely to draw our attention to this important point. K.N. Mathur also has included affiliation of remedies to the specific organs in his "Systematic Materia Medica". Physiological action of remedies and their specific action on the specific organs of the body have been discussed in detail in William H. Burt's "Physiological Materia Medica".

Some remedies have very peculiar affinity with particular parts of the body. This is why ascertaining the exact location and finding the remedy accordingly is, sometimes, very necessary. Farrington says,

"You will find that Natrum carb. will relieve soreness of the feet, and particularly of the soles, accompanied by swelling of those parts. You may also use it for ulcers on or about the heels after a long walk. This symptom brings to mind a peculiar circumstance that I would like to mention. Certain remedies have an affinity for certain parts of the body. A soldier who had been marching a great deal had two ulcers, one on the heel, the other on the instep. Natrum carb. cured the one on the heel but not the one on the instep, which was afterwards cured by Lycopodium. LYCOPODIUM acts on the instep and Natrum carb. on the heel. The same thing you note all over the body. There are drugs that act on the right tonsil and not at all on the left. You find some remedies which act on the great toe and not at all on the others."

(Farrington, Clinical Materia Medica, P. 847)

However this is rarely the case and the basic principle is always totality of symptoms in which general symtopms paly an important role.

Although in Homoeopathic practice we do not need to go very deep into the pathological condition and laboratory findings, yet the disease action of medicines is definitely not negligible. A Homoeopath should be well aware of every aspect of each medicine and must give due importance to every aspect in the selection of Homoeopathic remedies.

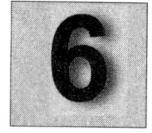

SYMPTOMS

Before going into the details of different types of symptoms we should understand what exactly symptoms are?

Yasgur's "Homoeopathic Dictionary" defines 'symptom' as,

"The phenomena of disease which lead to complaints on the part of the ill person".

(Jay Yasgur, Homoeopathic Dictionary P. 245)

He also highlights the difference between symptoms and signs,

"Signs and symptoms are the only perceptible form of disease ('dysfunctional vital force'), and their full comprehension is necessary to intelligently understand the patient's loss of well-being. A sign is generally understood to be objective (red stripe down the middle of the tongue, fever, sweating, etc.) while a symptom is subjective and conveys how the patient feels, e.g. " my leg hurts" is a symptom, albeit not very good one."

(Jay Yasgur, Homoeopathic Dictionary P. 245)

Stuart Close in "The Genius of Homoeopathy" defines 'symptom' more clearly with reference to Hahnemann,

"In general, a symptom is any evidence of disease, or change from a state of health. In materia medica no relevant fact is too insignificant to be overlooked. There is a place and use for every fact, for science has learned that "Nature never trifles." A symptom which appears trifling to the careless or superficial examiner may become, in the hands of the expert, the key which unlocks a difficult problem in therapeutics.

Hahnemann defines symptoms broadly as, "any manifestation of a deviation from a former state of health, perceptible by the patient, the individuals around him or the physician".

(Stuart Close, The Genius of Homoeopathy PP.149-50)

So any deviation from a former state of health is called a 'symptom' whether it has been produced in the individual by the influence of a disease or a drug or some other particular cause. Materia medica is a record of symptoms produced in healthy human beings by the influence of medicines.

In fact symptoms of a medicine described in the materia medica are the real source to recognize it and to make its selection in any case. But every remedy has numerous symptoms and it is not true that the selection can be made on any one or two of all the symptoms. Such a selection would not lead to a successful prescription. Rather nearly in every case there are certain basic and indispensable symptoms and a remedy selected on such important symptoms can bring a cure. Certainly if the basic and fundamental symptom of the patient, on which the whole disease is based, would be missing in the selected remedy it would not cause a complete cure. Thus before studying Materia Medica we must know thoroughly what kind of symptoms (either in the remedy or in the patient) are fundamentally important? What kind of symptoms should be the basis of a Homoeopathic prescription? Unless we know the classification, gradation and ranking of symptoms thoroughly we cannot adopt exact mode of studying the Materia Medica in order to master it and bring it to its fuller use. Stuart Close says,

"Knowledge of the true nature and constitution of a symptom is necessary in proving or testing medicines; in the examination of a patient; in the study of the materia medica and in the selection and management of the indicated remedy."

(Stuart Close, The Genius of Homoeopathy P.149)

Basically symptoms are divided into two kinds:
1. General Symptoms
2. Particular Symptoms

GENERAL SYMPTOMS

Symptoms that concern the whole patient, that are related to the individual in general; conditions existing in, or situations affecting the patient in general, are all General Symptoms e.g. anger, irritability, malice, (jealousy), company desire, company aversion, intolerance of or desire for heat or cold, eating after aggravation or amelioration in the aggregate, sexual desire/passion increased or diminished, most or all symptoms better or worse after sleep etc. Yasgur's "Homoeopathic Dictionary" defines General Symptom as,

"One which encompasses the whole person; the 'I' symptom: "I feel better in the cold weather/while walking/after a nap." These are symptoms which pertain to and characterize the whole person. Dreams come under this heading only if a dream is repeated over and over."

(Jay Yasgur, Homoeopathic Dictionary P.250)

Importance of General Symptoms

"Put your patient, as a whole, in order, and he will straighten out the disorder of his parts. You have got to get at him; and you can only get at him through his general and mental symptoms."

(Repertorizing: Margaret Tyler and John Weir, Kent's Repertory P.6)

General symptoms are the basic, collective and true indications, exhibitions and proclamations of the internal disordered state—the disorders of vital force. Hence we should mostly pay attention to General Symptoms either in taking the case or studying Materia Medica. On account of their importance Hahnemann especially draws our attention to the General Symptoms (§ 88, 211, 212, 213). Those who understand the status and importance of General Symptoms could practice Homoeopathy successfully and those who do not understand these, in spite of adopting Homoeopathy could not practice it well. They use Homoeopathic dilutions but because their prescriptions are not based on fundamental General Symptoms, they cannot achieve attractive and conspicuous results. Their cures, even perfect ones, are only accidental because they themselves do not know what the reasons were behind their cures or failures. Why does a remedy sometimes cause a very brilliant cure and at another time absolute failure?

We must always keep in mind that the part (e.g. an organ) is always dependant on the integrity of the whole (the entire person). In other words the minority is dependant on the majority. Similarly every organ is dependent on the whole organism. An organ cannot live apart from man. If it is so, how can it become diseased without a diseased condition in the whole? It is always said that the child is sick because there is infection in the tonsils or throat and that one is sick because of cholilithiasis or the enlargement of the heart. The question is, if a child's tonsils suppurate after getting cold, did the cold touch only the tonsils? No, rather the cold affected the child as a whole and there is a condition in the child of being sick after getting cold and the disease has centered itself in the throat or chest. An organ cannot become diseased without a disordered state of the whole man. Man gets sick; his vital force is sick and weak, which equally exists in the whole man, not less or more in any of its parts. If we wish to restore the health of an organ we must restore the health of vital force whose weakness and disorder is the basic reason of the sickness. If a child's chest is affected by cold we shall have to reinstate all the system that has been affected by the cold. Removing the gall bladder neither repairs the altered functions that are causing damage to the gall bladder or liver, nor restores the patient to health. If we wish to make a true cure we have to put in order the functions that are, in fact, making these gallstones; we shall have to repair that disordered state of the organism which has resulted in disease and misery.

That is why Hahnemann especially has drawn our attention to General Symptoms. Without considering General Symptoms in the case, we would really overlook the full usefulness of Homoeopathy. A sick organ will remain sick if we do not cure the person as a whole. How can we repair a part without curing the disordered state on the whole (General symptoms)? If in the details given by the patient or his relatives/friends there is no information about the main functions of the body or about the mental and physical conditions, we must question these in order to have a fuller picture of the disease.

That is to say, due to the disease or along with the disease, all changes in the mental and physical spheres and all changes in the main functions of the body are essential components of the disease that we should understand. This will provide us with a complete knowledge of the disease. In Homoeopathic parlance, if in the details provided by the patient there are only Particular Symptoms we must acquire all General Symptoms and choose a remedy that includes them all. Hahnemann says in Aphorism No. 88

"If in these voluntary details nothing has been mentioned respecting several facts or functions of the body or his mental state, the physician asks what more can be told in regard to these parts and these functions or the state of his disposition or mind, but in doing this he only makes use of general expressions, in order that his information may be obliged to enter into special details concerning them."

(Hahnemann, Organon, Aphorism No. 88, P. 175)

Types of General Symptoms

(a) Mental/Emotional Symptoms

Hahnemann emphasized the symptoms of the mind, hence we see how clearly the master comprehended the importance of the direction of symptoms; the more interior first, the mind, the exterior last, the physical or bodily symptoms.

(Kent, Lesser Writings P. 463)

Among the Generals, the symptoms of the first grade are, if well marked, the MENTAL SYMPTOMS. These take the highest rank: and a strongly marked mental symptom will always rule out any number of poorly marked symptoms of lesser grade.

(Margaret Tyler and John Weir, Repertorizing, Kent's Repertory P. 3)

If well marked, mental symptoms are of the highest grade and importance in Homoeopathic prescribing. If a person has a well-marked mental symptom of a drug and a well-marked absolute symptom of another, the drug with the mental symptom takes precedence over the other.

(Garth Boericke, Principles of Homoeopathy P. 48)

Mind is the inner most element of man. All functions in the man, either voluntary or involuntary (Intentional or unintentional) befall from inner to outer. When man intends or plans any thing, first of all its design arises in the mind. Then plan or order transfers to the nerves and afterward organs or parts perform that task in subjection to the nerves. If there is no order from the mind or if it has been suspended, everything will be suspended even if all other organs seem to be physically well. The Vital Force is equally present in man's entirety. When the vital force is disordered and unbalanced, a disordered state exists in the entire person and as a result changes take place on different levels and parts. So in Homoeopathy, changes that take place in the the central, basic and important parts/levels are logically considered central, basic and important changes. Farrington says,

"You go on collecting these symptoms, both subjective and objective. If you are skilled in the analysis of the excreta of the body, you should make use of your knowledge to determine the elimination of urates, phosphates etc. These are facts and, in their places, are invaluable. I would have you mind this expression, IN THEIR PLACE VALUABLE, OUT OF PLACE VALUELESS AND EVEN HARMFUL. An increase in the elimination of urea would weigh nothing in the balance, against the mental state. All symptoms of the Materia Medica are not of the same value. They are relative in value."

(Farrington, Clinical Materia Medica, P. 4)

Since all the functions in man befall from inner to outer and always go on happening this way, if we try to repair the external parts disregarding the internal changes there will always be failure. If there seems some betterment it will be temporary and internal disorder will go on to alter the externals also. If the internal disorder is incorrectly suppressed then that will travel to some deeper level in the organism. Therefore in every disease we must acquire the internal, central and important symptoms with great attention. Hahnemann says,

> § 211 "This holds good to such an extent, that the state of the disposition of the patient often chiefly determines the selection of the homoeopathic remedy, as being a decidedly characteristic symptom which can least of all remain concealed from the accurately observing physician".
>
> *(Hahnemann, Organon, P. 249)*
>
> § 212 "The Creator of therapeutic agents has also had particular regard to this main feature of all diseases, the altered state of the disposition and mind, for there is no powerful medicinal substance in the world which does not very notably alter the state of the disposition and

mind in the healthy individual who tests it, and every medicine does so in a different manner".

(Hahnemann, Organon, P. 249)

§ 213 "We shall, therefore, never be able to cure conformably to nature - that is to say, homoeopathically - if we do not, in every case of disease, even in such as are acute, observe, along with the other symptoms, those relating to the changes in the state of the mind and disposition, and if we do not select, for the patient's relief, from among the medicines a disease-force which, in addition to the similarity of its other symptoms to those of the disease, is also capable of producing a similar state of the disposition and mind."

(Hahnemann, Organon, PP. 249-50)

The second reason for considering the mental symptoms most important is that Homoeopathic remedies have been evidently proved to produce changes on mental/emotional levels and when such symptoms are available in patients, the selection of the remedy is achieved with confidence. The more knowledge and attention we have of mental symptoms in the Materia Medica the easier it is to obtain these symptoms from the patients.

Although necessary, it is not always easy to elicit these symptoms as most patients do not notice characteristics of themselves at mental/emotional levels. Or the patients do not realize they are related to their disease. In other cases the patients do not wish to share their personal affairs with the physician. Nevertheless with experience and continuous diligence the Homoeopathic physician can subtly obtain the necessary information.

Some mental symptoms are more important than others. Experts have divided mental faculty into three parts.

(1) Will   (2) Intellect/understanding   (3) Memory

Whenever we start learning something, first of all it comes to the memory then into intellect and after that into the will. For instance, when we learn driving, firstly we memorize the names and functions of all parts of the car. We memorize this is such thing and performs such a function, and we have to use such a thing for such a purpose. It means that learning has come to the memory (the outer layer of mind). And when we start driving we understand the function of every part of the car, everything memorized comes into the intellect and understanding (the middle layer of mind). Afterwards a time comes when we are talking to some one on a very serious subject or listing to music while driving the car. That is to say now we don't need to use our memory and understanding to drive the car. Now we drive automatically which means that learning has come into the will, into the intention (the inner most of mind). And when something goes out of the mind it goes in the reverse order.

Therefore, symptoms related to will, intention, behavior and mental desires and aversions are the most valuable, the supreme symptoms. Such as Company Desire or Aversion, Irritability, Obstinate, Malice, Suspiciousness, Anger, Timidity, Indolence, Changes in Behavior, Sensitiveness and Fears etc. Symptoms related to intellect and understanding have second grade in mental symptoms e.g. comprehension difficult, confusion of mind, and all kinds of delusions etc. ---- the disorders of intellect and understanding. Symptoms that belong to memory have third grade in mental symptoms such as weakness of memory, forgetfulness and different disorders of the memory. These are the less important mental symptoms.

(b) Physical General Symptoms

Along with the mental and psychic symptoms, Hahnemann teaches us to obtain information about the changes in the conditions and states that concern the whole body.

"Second in grade, after mental symptoms, and his reactions to mental environment, come, if well marked, such general symptoms of the patient as his reactions, as a whole, to bodily environment: --- to times and seasons, to heat and cold, to damp and dry, to storm and tempest, to position, pressure, motion, jar, touch, etc.

(Margaret Tyler and John Weir, Repertorizing, Kent's Repertory, P. 4)

George Vithoulkas in "The Science of Homoeopathy" describes Physical General Symptoms as,

"There are also physical general symptoms. These refer to physical states which apply to the person as whole, the patient may say, "I feel very cold all the time" or "I cannot tolerate the Sun," or "I am always tired".

(George Vithoulkas, The Science of Homoeopathy, P.194)

So the physical General symptoms relate to the factors that influence all of the body. They physically affect the whole body, such as cold, heat, motion, exertion, or change of weather etc. That is to say what are the effects of cold or heat on the whole body; do all the symptoms get worse or better by motion, lying, pressure, or touch? What are the effects of weather on the body as a whole? These are a few examples. In Kent's Repertory an extensive chapter (Generalities) has been reserved for Physical General Symptoms, states and modalities that can be used as General Symptoms. After mentals, these are the most important symptoms being related to the whole body. A remedy can produce good effects on the whole body if it is similar to the whole of it. If a remedy is similar to particular symptoms and dissimilar to physical generals how can it touch the disease on physical general level and how can it cause changes on the whole and bring a complete cure?

(c) Food Symptoms

Next to mental and physical generals, very important are the symptoms that occur by means of the stomach yet are related to the entire body. Such as abnormal conditions of appetite or thirst, longing or loathing of different foods and drinks, aggravation or amelioration by any kind of food in the most or all of symptoms etc. For example a patient has an extreme thirst. Now the thirst occurs in stomach and is felt in the mouth and throat but in the extreme thirst if he cannot find water he will suffer wholly and by drinking it, he will get satisfied physically as well as mentally. Moreover water affects the whole body. There are effects of eating and drinking on the whole body. So extreme longing or loathing of different food items or aggravation or amelioration by them in collective symptoms are considered General Symptoms. Such symptoms also facilitate the selection of Homoeopathic remedy. Vithoulkas says,

"Even food cravings or aversions are considered physical general symptoms: "I crave sweets, "I hate meat," or "I am always thirsty for cold drinks". These symptoms represent manifestation of the entire organism, and not merely of stomach."

(George Vithoulkas, The Science of Homoeopathy, P.194)

But in obtaining these general symptoms (occurring by means of stomach) and ranking them in the totality of symptoms we shall be careful because merely liking or disliking of any edible thing would not be a symptom. Liking and disliking of these things may be a little different in every individual but if an individual has a strong desire or aversion then it will definitely be a general symptom.

"The third-grade General symptoms are the food CRAVINGS AND AVERSIONS. But to be elevated to such rank, they must not be mere likes and dislikes, but longings and loathings".

(Margaret Tyler and John Weir, Repertorizing, Kent's Repertory, P.5)

Also if there is an aggravation or amelioration in the most or all symptoms by any of these things it will be considered one of general symptoms or a general modality. While symptoms occurring from stomach and limited to it, are particular symptoms such as pain in stomach, heartburn, eructations, hiccough etc. Symptoms coming from stomach and concerning the whole man are always generals.

(d) Sex Symptoms

The next generals are the sexual symptoms. Such as nymphomania, diminished sexual desire, aggravation or amelioration during or after coition in most or all symptoms; symptoms collectively or mostly worse or better before, during or after menses etc. In these symptoms also only those are generals that are related to the whole person. If a symptom is limited merely to sexual organs that would not be a general one, such as leucorrhoea, menses scanty or profuse, itching on genital parts, eruptions, quick ejaculation, erection incomplete, dysmenorrhoea, spermatorrhoea, nightly emissions etc. Nevertheless if most or all symptoms are better or worse during or after menses, or they are agg. or amel. before during or after coitus then they affect man as a whole and are therefore generals. In "The Science of Homoeopathy" Vithoulkas says,

"Sex symptoms are considered next in importance to physical general symptoms. They include such things as the degree of sexual desire, the degree of sexual satisfaction, and aggravation and amelioration from menses. Such symptoms having to do with the particular genital organs, however, are listed as local symptoms: i.e., discharges, menstrual irregularities, or inability to develop or maintain an erection."

(George Vithoulkas, The Science of Homoeopathy, P.194)

(e) Sleep Symptoms

Since sleep happens in the mind and the mind is the center of man, symptoms of sleep that concern the whole man are also considered general symptoms . For instance, aggravation or amelioration. during or after sleep in most or all symptoms, positions during sleep or dream etc.

"Of next importance are sleep symptoms, which, of course, are general symptoms. They arise out of mental and emotional states, certain hormonal and electromagnetic imbalances, physical restlessness, etc. thus we list such symptoms as the position in which the patient sleeps, positions in which it is impossible to sleep or in which disturbing dreams occur, parts of the body which tend to be uncovered during sleep, times of waking, sleeplessness, sleepiness, etc."

(George Vithoulkas, *The Science of Homoeopathy*, P.194)

(f) Chief Complaint

The Chief Complaint for which the patient consults us is also considered important like General Symptoms. H.A.Roberts says,

"In chronic work it is necessary to take into consideration the General Symptoms. By general symptoms we mean those symptoms which pertain to the patient as a whole, or to the complaint which he brings to us."

(H.A. Roberts, *Principles and Art of Cure by Homoeopathy*, P. 80)

Some experts, like Kent, do not include the chief complaint in general symptoms unless it belongs to their above mentioned types. Of course a patient's chief complaint may be a general as well as a particular symptom. We can settle the matter in this way that if a patient's chief complaint is a particular symptom it should be considered more important than other mere particulars.

(g) Pathological General Symptoms (Pathological Predispositions or Tendencies)

Tendency to catch cold, haemorrhagic tendency, tendency to skin affections or suppurations, hereditary miasmatic tendencies etc. are also considered important like general symptoms. Some Kentian homoeopaths do not consider the chief complaint or pathological tendencies as generals. But this is a mistake. I also made the same mistake in early years of my practice and faced many failures due to it. Some times a pathological condition is so dominant that we cannot do anything for the patient unless we select a medicine that has a definite action on that pathology. We see a lot of pathological conditions in "Generalities" chapter of Kent's repertory. For instance: apoplexy, atrophy of glands, blackness of external parts, cancerous affections, caries of bones, catalepsy, chlorosis, chorea, congestion of blood, convulsions, cyanosis, distention of blood vessels, dropsy, emaciation, fistulae of glands, hemorrhage, heat flushes, induration of glands, inflammation, mucous secretions increased and so on.

Rajan Sankaran says,

"We can call these symptoms the pathological generals, or the pathological tendencies of a given remedy. And my mind will only be fully satisfied when the pathological generals match between the remedy and the patient.

For example in Valeriana, the first sentence in Phatak's Materia Medica is "Mental and physical dispositions change suddenly, and go to extremes." He is saying that the grand generalization is very quick change.

Suppose a patient has a haemorrhagic tendency. Then you look for remedies that have haemorrhage as a pathological general. In another patient, you see a tendency to collapse. Here collapse becomes the pathological general, and you think of remedies like Carbo vegetabilis and Veratrum album where collapse is prominent.

Now suppose I have case in which the patient has fear of dark, fear to be alone, fears of this and that, and it looks like Calcarea carbonica. But when I asked what happens with the fear, the patient says that she becomes completely stupefied, that she cannot do any thing. For a few minutes nothing can happen, almost as if she is paralyzed. This symptom is called 'catalepsy'. I will first look to see which remedies have this tendency to catalepsy. And now I see that it does not look like Calcarea carbonica, because that remedy does not have catalepsy in its nature. So the basic nature of the pathology has to match, as well as the Family, Kingdom, Miasm and Characteristic Symptoms.

Every remedy has such pathological generals, and they are usually given in the first few lines in both Phatak's Materia Medica and Boger's Synoptic Key. In Boger it is especially clear. For example, in Opium the pathological general is painlessness, insensibility, numbness. If I see the pathology or the complaint of the patient has to do with numbness or insensibility, one of remedies that I think of is Opium.

Rubrics for pathological generals are very easily found in Phatak's Repertory. Examples are: 'Calculi, formation of'; 'Neuralgia'; 'Haemorrhage'; 'Numbness'; 'Venosity'; 'Collapse'; 'Convulsion'; 'Cancer'; 'Paralysis'. And there are many more.

These are characteristic pathologies at the general level, and the most important remedies for those tendencies are given there. If you go to Kent and to larger repertories you will be lost because a much greater range of remedies is given. Thus Phatak's Repertory is best to use when you have a pathological general and you want to know the main remedies that have that kind of pathology. For example in Lyssin the main pathology is spasm, with high acute sense. In Laurocerosus, the pathological general is sudden debility and collapse. Secale Cornutum has haemorrhage and gangrene."

(Rajan Sankaran, The Synergy in Homoeopathy, PP. 107-8)

In short all symptoms related to the patient on the whole or his most organs and parts are general and fundamentally important for the selection of medicine. A general curative action of a homoeopathic remedy depends on these General Symptoms.

Therefore we should always be very attentive to the general symptoms in the study of Materia Medica; firstly because cure cannot be achieved if general symptoms are not similar in the patient and the remedy. Secondly general symptoms are prominent and definite. Such symptoms are easy to attain and retain in the mind. When we are well familiar with these basic and important symptoms of every remedy we can easily recognize the most appropriate Homoeopathic remedy for every patient. Thirdly, particular symptoms resemble each other and cannot help us in individualizing and differentiating--- the process for the choice of a remedy. General symptoms are mostly different. They help us in arriving at the most suitable Homoeopathic remedy. For instance, a patient is presenting with Hemorrhoids. But on the basis of Hemorrhoids only we cannot select a correct homoeopathic remedy. However when all general symptoms such as mentals, sensitivity to heat and cold and all others are before us, the most suitable Homoeopathic remedy will be marked out clearly.

PARTICULAR SYMPTOMS

Symptoms related to one part or some particular organ of the body are called particular symptoms viz headache, conjunctivitis, pain in the knee, or Haemorrhoids etc. It has already been expalined that particular symptoms being limited and smaller have less importance. Since they resemble each other very much, they hardly help us in individualization. However if a particular symptom is equally affecting most parts of the body, it will become as important as a general symptom. For example if a patient has burning pain in any part of the body along with burning or burning pains in other parts also, then burning pain will be one of his general symptoms and his remedy will be selected from medicines having this symptom.

"Great mistakes may come from going too deep into particulars before the generals are settled. Any army of soldiers without the line of officers could not be but a mob; such a mob of confusion is our materia medica to the man who has not the command".

(Kent, Lesser Writings, P.466)

"And now, at last, you come to the PARTICULARS---the symptoms that bulk so largely for the patient, and for which he is as the matter of fact, actually consulting. You will have taken them down first, with the utmost care and detail, listening to his story, and interrupting as little as possible ; but you will consider them last : for these symptoms are really of minor importance from your point of view (certainly in chronic cases) because they are not general to the patient as a living whole, but only particulars to some part of him."

(Margaret Tyler and John Weir, Repertorizing, Kent's Repertory, P. 5)

"Physical particular symptoms are given relatively minor significance. Even though such symptoms may be of great intensity, they affect only a part of the organism and are therefore a relatively insignificant manifestation of the defense mechanism."

(G. Vithoulkas, The Science of Homoeopathy, P. 194)

"Particular/local symptoms: referring to a part of the body or to the disease. These symptoms are generally less important than the generals unless they are peculiar. 'My head aches' is a useless particular symptom, but if the symptom is 'My head aches only between 10 AM and 2 PM', this is peculiar (even strange and rare) and indicates Nat-Mur."

(Jay Yasgur, Homoeopathic Dictionary, P. 252)

Difference between Particular Symptoms and Localized Peculiar Sensations

An important point in relation to particular symptoms is that we should not mix them with localized peculiar sensations such as sensation as if "something were alive in head (Crot-t, Sil)", sensation of "fish-bone or splinter in throat", sensation as if "there were something alive in abdomen" or sensation as if "legs were made of wood or glass". Such symptoms, though localized, are peculiar sensations that often help us in arriving at required remedy. Yasgur's "Homoeopathic Dictionary" differentiates local/ particular symptoms form localized peculiar sensations as under,

"Locals are symptoms associated just with the chief complaint. For example, a patient is seen for hip pain. He describes his symptoms as better with motion, worse on wet, humid days, with lancinating pains upon lying on the right side and a warmth which seems to radiate from the painful area. These are symptoms directly associated with the hip and are termed local. Some may refer to local symptoms as particulars. Do not confuse local symptoms with localized sensations. Sensations and localized sensations, if pronounced enough, may act as keynotes/leaders steering you to the correct remedy. For example, the symptom 'lancinating pains in the sacrum on stooping, extending into the buttocks' is a localized sensation."

(Jay Yasgur, Homoeopathic Dictionary, P. 251)

"These localized sensations, however, are local/particular symptoms and are less important than the rare and uncommon general symptoms. H.A. Robert says in the foreword of his "Sensations as if",

"Let the single symptom be only a partial indication to the application of the materia medica. Beware the keynote that is not backed up by knowledge of, or reference to, the materia medica. No single symptoms, no matter how "strange, rare and peculiar", can stand without the support of well taken case, and the likeness of the whole patient to the remedy".

(H.A. Robert, Sensations as if, Foreword)

PATHOLOGICAL SYMPTOMS

Ultimate pathological and organic/tissue changes are called Pathological Symptoms such as tonsillitis, haemorrhoids, fistula, eczema, otorrhoea etc. Laboratory findings and results of different lab tests also belong to this group. Yasgur defines pathological symptoms as,

"An objective expression of the disease, such as hypertension, anemia, fibrillation, bleeding, fever, profuse watery diarrhea".

(Jay Yasgur, Homoeopathic Dictionary, P. 253)

Vithoulkas reflects on this group of symptoms as under,

"Finally, of least significance are pathological tissue changes. These have tremendous importance for making an allopathic diagnosis, and also for determining a prognostic impression, but they are relatively unimportant for the actual selection of a remedy. For example, the common problem of delayed urination in an elderly man with an enlarged prostate gland cannot be used for homoeopathic purposes".

(George Vithoulkas, The Science of Homoeopathy P. 194)

Usually patients consult the physician for pathological symptoms but these are the least important for a homoeopathic selection of medicine. These are mostly common and diagnostic symptoms that do not help us in individualization.

Some people, being unaware of the principles, make their selections on the basis of these pathological symptoms such as Calc-s or Silicea for suppurations, Aesculis and Collinsonia for hemorrhoids etc. But this is very dangerous. Often pathological symptoms are suppressed by such selections. Whereas the disease goes on developing inwardly and at last becomes fatal. A homoeopathic physician brought to me a case of another homoeopath. He had bone fractures in an accident and his wounds were suppurating. He started taking Calc-s in low potencies. It stopped the pus but he was caught by some severe physical and mental symptoms. Calc-s had been prescribed on pathological symptoms but it was not similar to the totality of the patient. Thus it suppressed the symptoms and the disease was metastasized to deeper levels. Recently I have seen a case of paralysis which started from paresis of tongue. Causticum was applied and it benefited many times when the complaint relapsed. The patient and her doctor were happy because they were able to solve the problem. But the result of this suppression was complete paralysis of the right side. This would never have happened if Causticum had been the correct remedy. If it were similar to the totality of the patient it would have rooted out the disease. Similarly hemorroids are suppressed by Nux-v. But if it is not thoroughly indicated the result is never favorable. Farrington says,

"In haemorrhoids, Nux may be useful when there is itching, keeping the patient awake at night, and frequently so severe as to compel the patient to sit in a tub of cold water for relief. There is frequent ineffectual urging to stool. There is bleeding from the piles. Unless Nux is thoroughly indicated, it should not be prescribed, for while, in such cases, it may cure the piles, it will excite some other trouble more unbearable than the one it has relieved."

(Farrington, Clinical Materia Medica, P. 208)

Once a homoeopath, who is a government employee, told me that he cured very chronic nasal catarhh of his officer with Sulphur 1M. He was completely free from catarrh which he had from many years. After some time the officer suffered from hemorrhoids. Again he cured him with a dose of Nux-v 1M. Then unfortunately the officer was caught by stomach ulcer. This time he didn't ask this homoeopath for medicine; if he had asked he would have cured him. I told in my heart. Yes you would have cured him of his life. The miserable homoeopath and the patient! The homoeopath only suppressed the conditions and metastasized the same.

In this way homoeopathic medicines also suppress pathological symptoms. This is more dangerous than allopathic suppressions because homoeopathic medicines are very deep and they metastasize the disease to deeper levels. Along with suppression of pathological ones other symptoms, necessary to know for homoeopathic treatment, also change and the case becomes very difficult, if not incurable.

A same pathological symptom, in different cases, may be result of different causes. For instance, Azospermia/ Oligospermia may be due to suppression of Gonorrhoea for which often Medorrhinum or Thuja serve curatively; it may be due to excessive masturbation in adolescence when sex organs are not fully developed; it also may be due to inherited syphilis. I have also seen psoric patients suffering from this problem who were cured by antipsoric remedies like Calc-c and Sulph etc. Another case of this pathology, in my record-book, that had signs of sycosis in his family, was cured by Silicea.

Abnormal position of fetus in last months of pregnancy is also a pathological condition. Some people give here Pulsatilla. Of course some cases are solved by it but some others not. Definitely cases that need other remedies would not be solved by Puls. A large number of these cases are solved by good homoeopaths with the help of different remedies like Arg-n, Bry, Carb-v, Merc, Puls and Sulph etc. indicated by the totality of symptoms. Abnormal position of fetus in Puls is due to excess of amniotic fluid; in Bry due to constipation and pressure of intestine toward uterus; in Carb-v due to pressure of gas accumulated in stomach and intestines. That is, a same pathological condition or symptoms may be due to many different causes/factors and along with varied general symptoms. When we apply the remedy similar to the totality, then the patient gets rid of all symptoms and is cured.

On seeing a few drops of pus we cannot determine from which part of the body the pus is coming out. A handkerchief wet by sweat does not tell us which region of the body was perspiring. A wart cut off the skin does not reveal on what part it was grown. Blood itself can never tell it has come from the nose, uterus or rectum. When these pathological things tell us nothing important, we should not base our prescriptions on them.

Pathologicals are common symptoms of diagnostic character that do not lead us to the required remedy. It has been told before that abnormal thirst, appetite, weakness and frequent urination are diagnostic symptoms of diabetes. These symptoms are not as valuable in a diabetic patient as in patients suffering from other diseases. We, as homoeopaths, should have knowledge of diagnostic symptoms of all diseases. But according to Kent we should know them but not to use them as the basis of our Homoeopathic selections. Gunavante quotes Kent as,

"It is necessary to know them. All become acquainted with diagnosis and pathology in order not to prescribe for the disease . . . If the physician does not know what the common symptoms are, i.e. what symptoms represent the various diseases, he will mistake of trying to fit remedy to such symptoms. The symptoms common to Bright's disease are dropsy, albumin in urine, weakness and the disturbed heart action. Any physician who would pretend to prescribe on these would show a great folly. The remedies that have produced such a complex of symptoms are very numerous."

(Gunavante, Introduction to Homoeopathic Prescribing P. 50)

Kent says in his "Lesser Writings",

"The more accurate the diagnosis and the more substantial its basis, the more inaccurate the prescription that is based upon it. The diagnosticians are the poorest prescribers, yet, in spite of all this, no harm can come from the finest sagacity in naming diseases. It must be understood, however, that the diagnosis does not reveal the nature of a disease in a manner to image a remedy. The diagnosis is the name of ultimates and exteriors, while it is the interior nature that must be perceived through the peculiar, characterizing signs and symptoms, in order to discover the remedy that will cure."

(J.T. Kent, Lesser Writings, P. 266)

But this does not mean we should select medicines which have no relation to the pathology of the patient at hand or we should avoid remedies that correspond to pathological symptoms. The best selected remedy is similar to all general, particular and pathological symptoms. Kent emphasizes only not to base the selection on pathological ones. We should depend on generals because they individualize and lead us to the decisive selection. We may say that pathological symptoms are paths or roads that mostly resemble each other and general symptoms are traffic signs and milestones. We are guided by milestones and traffic signs and walk on the road to reach our destination. We individualize by generals, match particulars and pathologicals to them and arrive at the best suited remedy. We can ignore pathologicals only when we have two remedies of which one is similar to Generals and the other to Pathologicals. Gunavante, in his "Introduction to Homoeopathic Prescribing" explains this point with reference to Gibson Miller as under,

"Finally, here is a gem from Gibson Miller's 'Comparative Value of symptoms'. After affirming at page 5, Hahnemann's directive that our main reliance should be placed almost exclusively on the peculiar and characteristic symptoms of the patient and not on those that are common to the disease. Miller now gives (at page 7) an apparently contradictory advice that "it would be foolish to ignore the symptoms that signify the disease... for however helpful the peculiar symptoms may be, it is the totality of the symptoms that determines the choice." Let us see how he argues this point,

In the foregoing, stress has been laid on the supreme importance of paying the greatest attention to the symptoms that are peculiar to the patient, but it would be foolish to ignore the symptoms that signify the disease. They must indeed be taken into consideration, but subsequent to, and of much less value than, those that are predicated of the patient. In a very large number of cases no one remedy corresponds to all the peculiar symptoms, but three or four seem to have equal numbers of them, and of approximately the same value. In such a state of affairs the remedy that has also the common symptoms best marked must prevail. It must never be kept in mind that there must be a general correspondence between all the symptoms of the patient and those of the remedy, and however helpful the peculiar symptoms may be in calling attention to certain remedies, yet they are not the sole guides; for, after all, it is the totality of the symptoms that determines the choice."

(Gunavante, Introduction to Homoeopathic Prescribing, PP. 57-58)

In the beginning, when I had studied Kent's Materia and not his "Lesser Writigns" I thought, like many of beginners, that pathology has no concern with homoeopathic selection; the selection must be on general symptoms and that general symptoms can suffice for selection. As my study expanded, I came to understand that it was not true. Kent, who was a great advocate of generals, did not completely ignore pathological symptoms,

"The study of true pathology should be encouraged, and is essential to the science of Homoeopathy, and no homoeopathician has ever discouraged it. Pathology is any discourse upon disease; it is broad and all-embracing. The study of disease as manifested through subjective and objective symptoms a study of lesions or results of diseases as made known by physical inspections, etc., etc., down to morbid anatomy, all should be known by homoeopathician, with a full appreciation of the true value of all. The disease in its course, history, and every known manifestation should be considered that the individuality may appear in one grand picture".

(J.T. Kent, Lesser Writings, P. 480)

Farrington settles the dispute of pathology and symtopms in this way,

"The statement made against me is that we cannot know what changes are taking place except through symptoms, therefore if one begins to talk about altered tissue, he at once pollutes homeopathy. This is true and it is false. It is true if you take this altered tissue alone. It is not true if you regard this altered tissue as a manifestation of the change in the vital force. I cannot see how there can be a symptom which is not at least the result of a change of function. I do not mean that you must give Bryonia because it acts on serous membranes; I do not mean that you must give Aconite because it produces dry skin, heat, etc. I do not say that you shall give Belladonna because it produces hyperaemia of the brain and dilatation of the pupil; but I do say that these drugs produce these effects, and if these effects are not alterations in function what are they ? We can know changes in the vital forces only by results, and these results are symptoms."

(Farrington, Clinical Materia Medica, P. 3)

Following description of Kali Hydriodicum by Farrington makes us clearly understand how we need to combine pathological state with the totality,

"It is also called for when the hepatization is so extensive that we have cerebral congestion or even an effusion into the brain as the result of this congestion. Now, the symptoms in these cases are as follows: First, they begin with very red face, the pupils are more or less dilated, and the patient is drowsy; in fact, showing a picture very much like that of Belladonna. You will, in all probability, give that remedy, but it does no good. The patient grows worse, the breathing becomes more heavy, and the pupils inactive to light, and you know then that you have a serious serous effusion into the brain, which must be checked in a short time or the patient dies. Why did not Belladonna cure? He who would prescribe by the symptoms alone in this case would fail, because he has not taken the totality of the case. The trouble did not start in the brain. The cerebral symptoms are secondary to others. What, then, is the primary trouble? You put your ear to the patient's chest, and you find one or both lungs consolidated ; hence, the blood cannot circulate through the lungs as it should, and the different organs in the body become congested. So until you have proved that Belladonna has produced such a condition you cannot expect it to do any good."

(Farrington, Clinical Materia Medica, P. 879)

Conclusion: Combine the pathological symptoms with the general and peculiar symptoms. This is the totality of symptoms that Hahnemann taught us in aphorisms 84 to 104.

COMMON AND UNCOMMON SYMPTOMS

All general and particular symptoms are further divided into two kinds.

(a) Common Symptoms

(b) Uncommon/Strange and Rare Symptoms

Symptoms found in numerous remedies and diagnostic symptoms of different diseases are called common symptoms such as anger, irritability, sensitiveness to heat or cold, diminished appetite, weakness and sleeplessness etc. Or frequent urination, abnormal appetite, thirst and weakness in all diabetic patients.

"Common symptoms are those which are common to human experience and have a very large number of remedies listed in the Repertory. For example, the symptom Aversion to Company, while not uncommon in human experience, is listed in the Repertory as having been produced by 100 remedies! In evaluating symptoms, one must keep in mind which symptoms are truly representative of the defense mechanism of the patient, and which are merely common manifestations of the diagnostic category of the pathological entity."

(George Vithoulkas, The Science of Homoeopathy, P.193)

Whereas symptoms not found in many remedies, or that seem to be very strange are called uncommon and rare symptoms as company aversion yet dread of being alone, chilliness with desire to uncover and pain in throat while swallowing liquids and not when swallowing solid food.

Kent defines common symptoms as,

"Common symptoms are such as are pathognomonic of diseases and of pathology, and such as are common to many remedies and are found in large rubrics in our repertories; e.g., constipation; nausea; irritability; delirium; weeping; weakness; trembling; chill; fever; sweat".

(J.T. Kent, Lesser Writings, P. 473)

He also highlights the difference between common and uncommon symptoms as,

"However some of these common symptoms may become peculiar where their circumstances are peculiar; e.g., trembling at any time or at all times all over the body and the limbs is a strong and most troublesome symptom, but it is not peculiar nor uncommon. But trembling before a storm, or during stool, or before menses, or during urination, is rare and srange.

Weakness is also common if constant, but if it comes only before menses, or before stool, or during a storm, it is at once quite uncommon, and changes the view of the case.

Chilliness, if constant, is common to many people, and is a srong common general as it is predicted of the whole patient, but if it comes only before or during menses, before or during stool, or while urinating, or only when in bed in the night, or only while eating,---then it is strange and peculiar, or uncommon"

(J.T. Kent, Lesser Writings, PP. 473-74)

We always identify and recognize things by their special and differentiating attributes rather than their common qualities. Such as for identifying someone we say it is the person who has blue eyes, long or flat nose and hair long or curly instead of saying the person who has two eyes, one nose, two ears, and hair on the scalp. In the same manner we cannot recognize a remedy by means of symptoms found in numerous remedies. We can recognize a remedy by means of symptoms not found in any other or in a large number of remedies. That is why Hahnemann advises us to pay special attention to uncommon, characteristic and strange symptoms. They lead us quickly to the required remedy.

"The common symptoms, without the peculiar symptoms, may give a good understanding of a given case except for prescribing. Common symptoms alone will lead to failure of the prescription. We might as well attempt to prescribe for nervous dyspepsia, gastritis, jaundice, gallstone colic, enteritis, constipation, or a bilious temperament. The beginner often fails because he has secured only the common symptoms".

(J.T. Kent, Lesser Writings, P.476)

"It must now be seen that the physician who has in mind only the pathology as a basis for his prescription has only what is most common, and therefore has no view of the totality, and therefore violates the first principle of prescribing. He prescribes for results, for endings, and not for things first, not for causes."

(J.T. Kent, Lesser Writings, P.474)

"Learn well the anatomy, pathology, chemistry, diagnosis, and the symptoms and the course of every disease and all disease ultimates, that common symptoms may be quickly and certainly known.

By this means it will be easier to say what symptoms are not common to the case in hand, and thereby to perceive that all symptoms present in a given case which are not common must be uncommon and predicated (in general or particular) of the patient. These must be foremost in guiding to the remedy and the common symptoms may fall in, taking their place naturally where they belong in each individual case of sickness. When this method is mastered, prescribing becomes easy, with experience."

(J.T. Kent, Lesser Writings, P. 232)

"A symptom may be common to all cases of a certain disease, and therefore of no great use in picking out the individual remedy for a particular case of that disease; or it may be common to a very great number of drugs, and therefore indicate one of a large group of remedies only; and so of very little use in Repertorizing."

(M. Tyler and John Weir, Repertorizing, Kent's Repertory, P. 9)

"There are two classes of symptoms in every case of disease: first, those that pertain to the disease, that is, the common or diagnostic ones, and second, those that pertain to the patient. The advance cases that present gross pathology, the ultimates of the disease, present but few symptoms as such. If we refer to the materia medica we shall find that almost every leading remedy has these common or diagnostic symptoms, such as headache, indigestion, sleeplessness, fever, etc. When the symptoms are so common to many remedies, how can we differentiate between them for applying them to the sick individual patient? We cannot differentiate them. That is why we say that we cannot base our prescriptions on these common or diagnostic symptoms."

(S.M.Gunavante: Introduction to Homoeopathic Prescribing, P. 49)

When we come across uncommon, strange and rare symptoms in a patient we are bound to find a remedy with such symptoms to cure him. A symptom cannot develop without a particular mechanism in the system peculiar to it. When there is such a strange and rare symptom in a patient, no remedy can cure him without being similar to that one also. Very often, we see such uncommon, characteristic, rare and strange symptom in remedies as well as in the patients. M.L. Tyler says,

"Drugs elicit queer and characteristic symptoms, mental and physical, from their provings: and when these match the queer and characteristic symptoms, mental and physical, of sick persons, they cure. The nearer the correspondence is the more certain is the cure."

(M.L. Tyler, Homoeopathic Drug Pictures, P.77)

This is a special attribute of Homoeopathy to consider and regard all changes in the patient brought by disease and set a mode of treatment according to the collective picture of the disease whether certain symptoms seem to have a connection with the name of the disease or not, or seem to be very strange.

So according to all these details a mental uncommon and prominent symptom would be the most important and highest in rank whereas a particular common and mild symptom would be least important and lowest in rank. See this table.

Ranking of Symptoms				
Types of symptoms		Severe	Moderate	Mild
Psychic/Mental	Uncommon	1	2	3
	Common	4	5	6
Physical and other Generals	Uncommon	7	8	9
	Common	10	11	12
Particulars	Uncommon	13	14	15
	Common	16	17	18
Pathologicals	Common	19	19	19

In this table symptoms have been arranged from more important to less important in descending order. Mental symptoms have been put in the upper column as they are highest in rank. Physical and other general symptoms are in the second column because they are less important to mentals and more important to particular symptoms. Whereas particular symptoms have been placed into third column for they are less important to the above mental and general symptoms. Pathological symptoms are in the lowest column because they are lowest in rank.

Symptoms also have been divided into three levels (severe, moderate and mild) on the basis of their intensity. Thus we have such a set of symptoms from which we may weigh every individual symptom. The chart shows that mental symptoms are the most important of all; especially a mental uncommon symptom that is also severe/prominent will be our number 1 symptom---the most important and highest in rank. Similarly a mental uncommon and moderate (not so much severe) symptom would be 2nd in rank. That is, a mental uncommon and "mild" symptom would be less important to mental uncommon "severe" and "moderate" symptoms but more important to rest of all. In the third column a particular common symptom which bears 18th number is less important to above all. In the last column pathologicals that are always common symptoms bear 19th number. They are least important of all.

CONCOMITANT SYMPTOMS

Literal meaning of concomitant is "an accompanying or attendant condition, circumstance, or thing". So Concomitant Symptom is one that occurs simultaneously with or accompanies another symptom (especially the chief complaint). For example, headache during constipation, yawning with fever or blurred vision before or during headache etc. Being common or particular such symptoms alone (not associated with another) may not be valuable. But when such symptoms occur simultaneously with another symptom, they become peculiar even strange and rare symptoms that greatly help in finding the required remedy.

Yasgur's "Homoeopathic Dictionary" defines and explains concomitant symptom as under,

"One occurring with or co-existing with the chief complaint, whether in the same general area or at a removed location. For example, a throbbing headache accompanying acute diarrhea, or right molar tooth pain accompanying blurred vision are considered concomitant symptoms to the chief complaint of acute diarrhea and blurred vision. Often the patient does not consider such symptoms to be very important because they are not a great source of bother to him. Yet they are important to the selection of the remedy."

(Jay Yasgur, Homoeopathic Dictionary, P.248)

KEYNOTE SYMPTOMS

"There is another ism that destroys Hahnemann's teaching, viz., the misunderstood keynote system. This system appeals to the memory only. It does not train the mind to know the character of the remedies. It makes the memory hold only a few fragments of the remedy. It omits the nature of the remedy or the image of the patient, which was the soul of Hahnemann's teaching. If we omit from our thoughts this soul, this image, we omit all upon which a homoeopathic prescription rests, viz., the totality."

(J.T. Kent, Lesser Writings, P.327)

The clear and prominent symptoms of a remedy are called its keynote symptoms. "Homoeopathic Dictionary" defines them as,

"One which is so apparent, so clear, that it suggests a small group of remedies or even a single remedy. For example, pain in the right shoulder blade points to Chelidonium."

(Jay Yasgur, Homoeopathic Dictionary, P.250)

Keynote Symptoms are very helpful in finding or arriving at the required remedy. When a patient presents some keynote symptoms of a remedy, it immediately comes before us if we know the keynotes. But we cannot decide our selection on a keynote of a remedy because it may be found in other remedies also. Beware, while keynote symptoms guide us, sometimes they misguide also. If we concentrate too much on a keynote symptom, it may sway us to ignore other important symptoms of the case.

Some people habitually prescribe on keynotes. They blindly give Rhus-Tox on its keynote--- motion amelioration and first motion aggravation. Similarly Lycopodium is used for complaints of right side and Lachesis for that of left side. Merc-sol is frequently given for Aphthae and salivation during sleep. Selection on one symptom in this way is harmful. Since remedy is prescribed on one of its prominent symptoms, it often suppresses that symptom. But such suppression does not mean a cure. A symptom suppressed in this way often returns after less or more time. Every time the symptom returns the same remedy is repeated and the case goes on becoming deeper, longer and more complicated instead of being cured. Some times other symptoms of the unnecessarily repeated remedy develop in the patient and the case goes into a condition that is challenging even for an expert and experienced homoeopath. Kent says,

"Too often the remedy has been only similar enough to the superficial symptoms to change the totality and the image comes back altered, therefore resembling another remedy, which must always be regared as a misfortune, by which the case is sometimes spoiled, and the hand of the master may fail to correct the wrong done"

(J.T. Kent, Lesser Writings, P. 417)

He says on another place,

"A mistake in the first remedy nearly always means death, (in cases of Diphtharia) or at least it masks the case. It would be strange if you, who know much about the art of healing, could make the first prescription of a remedy so far from similar that it did not act. You know if it is similar at all it will make changes in that symptom image, and if it is similar enough it will cure; therefore you need not hope that if your first prescription did not cure it was so dissimilar it was harmless. You must expect to cure, or begin the cure with the first prescription; then all is easy, as the changes now observed are such as bring joy to the hearts of the family and to the doctor. You must, therefore, never prescribe on the first flitting evidences of the sickness, but according to the true saying: "First be sure you are right and then go ahead"

"The first prescription, when incorrectly chosen, will most likely change the symptoms, but the patient will go on from bad to worse and the next prescription must be a matter of guess-work, as the index has been spoiled, and hence the mortalities".

(J.T. Kent, Lesser Writings, PP. 279-80)

Vithoulkas says about cases spoiled by incorrect homoeopathic prescriptions,

"Patients who have already had years of homoeopathic treatment without significant benefit are those which cause any experienced homoeopath to cringe inwardly. They are the most dreaded of cases because they are the most difficult to treat."

(G. Vithoulkas, The Science of Homoeopathy, P.248)

I have dealt with case of a homoeopathic doctor who had been taking Arsenic Alb for restlessness and anxiety (a well known keynote symptom of the remedy). He started taking it from 30th potency and reached CM. But he was not cured because the selection was made on a keynote instead of the totality. Arsenic is also applied on its keynote: frequent thirst for small quantities. But when we consult Kent's Repertory for this symptom we see 19 remedies listed under this rubric. When a patient has this symptom any of the 19 may be his remedy and definitely the most similar to the totality will be the curative one. Merc is misused on its keynote symptoms of mouth and Farrington advises us to avoid such a misuse,

"With all these symptoms you find the tongue dark brown, and dry and cracked. The cracks gape considerably, and even bleed at times. Sometimes the tongue and mouth are covered with a brownish, tenacious mucus. At other times you find the tongue taking the imprint of the teeth. Now, let me beg of you not to give Mercurius simply because the later symtoptom is present. Mercurius has very little application to typhoid fever; it will spoil your case unless decided icteroid symptoms are present."

(Farrington, Clinical Materia Medica, P. 257)

Our renowned homoeopaths who had been using keynotes successfully knew the philosophy very well and were keen observer of the principles. They used keynotes only as a helping tool and prescribed according to the law, that is, according to the totality. Yasgur says,

"Keynotes are actually peculiar symptoms which have taken flavor and tend to point almost directly to a remedy, yet if keynotes are taken as final and the generals do not confirm them, failures often result. Many of the great homoeopathic prescribers (Lippe, Allen, Boger) were very successful keynote prescribers, but you must realize that they had keen 'totality perceptions' and thus would not allow false-positives to sway them"

(Jay Yasgur, Homoeopathic Dictionary, P.251)

Farrington says in his lecture on Cocculus,

"Now, whatever individual characteristics you may have for a drug in an individual case, these characteristics should agree with the general effects of the drug; otherwise, you are making a partial selection."

(Farrington, Clinical Materia Medica, P. 297)

SUBJECTIVE AND OBJECTIVE SYMPTOMS

Personal feelings and sensations of the patient that the physician and other bystanders cannot observe or detect are called Subjective Symptoms. For example, love, hatred, chilliness without shivering, pain, and its different kinds, longings and loathings etc. Symptoms that the physician and other bystanders can observe or detect by their senses are called Objective Symptoms such as fever, swelling, cough and perspiration etc.

Since subjective symptoms are personal feelings and sensations of the patient, they are considered internal and important symptoms of the case.

It is also said that patient describes subjective symptoms by 'I' such as "I feel better in cold air", "I am always thirsty", "I like sweets" or "I dislike fats" etc. Whereas objective symptoms are described by the phrase 'my' such as "my throat is sore", "my head aches" etc. But sometimes this is confusing. The patient may say "my appetite is not good", "my anger is violent". Now he is telling subjective symptoms but the phrase used is 'my'. So it is not important what phrase is being used but what is important is the kind of the symptom being described.

It is also said in relation to general and particular symptoms that general symptoms are described by 'I' whereas particulars by 'my'. But here again the phraseology may cause confusion because the patient may use opposite words. He may say "I am constipated", I cannot hold the urging for urine". These are particular symptoms narrated by phrase 'I'. On the other hand, "my sexual desire is increased", "my appetite is poor" are general symptoms described by phrase 'my'. So this phraseology is not basic. Basically we should understand to which thing the symptom belongs. If a symptom is limited to a single part or an organ, it is particular. Whereas one that belongs to the whole is general.

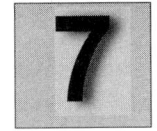

MODALITIES

Nash says,

"If Bœnninghausen had never done anything but given us his incomparable chapter on aggravations and ameliorations, this alone would have immortalised him."

(Nash, Leaders in Homoeopathic Therapeutics, P. 18)

Jay Yasgur in his "Homoeopathic Dictionary" defines Modality as under,

"A condition that makes the ill person or a particular symptom better or worse. A circumstance giving rise to an increase or decrease of a symptom. For instance the patient is worse (<) from wet weather, after midnight and cold drinks; or he is better (>) from heat, elevating the head and from warm/hot drinks. Modalities are helpful in choosing the correct remedy."

To define Modalities more clearly Yasgur quotes Garth Boericke as,

"Modalities are conditions which influence or modify drug action. The main group are time, temperature, weather, motion, menstruation, position, perspiration, eating and emotion. A particular point also is that there are two types of Modalities: 1) those that apply to the person as a whole, 2) those that apply to a person's particular complaint or involve an organ."

(Jay Yasgur, Homoeopathic Dictionary, PP.155-56)

This usual meaning does not express the real importance and usefulness of modalities in Homoeopathy practice.

That is why; many students and some Homoeopaths do not pay necessary attention to them and make mistakes in their selection. Consequently they face failures. I think if we ponder over the verbal meanings of "MODALITIES" we can understand their importance and usefulness well.

Verbal meanings of Modality as given in Oxford Dictionary are "the quality or fact of being modal, a modal quality or circumstance, the modal attributes of something." Where as "Modal" means "of or pertaining to or indicating a mode or mood"

Now Modalities of a remedy would mean to us "What is the mode or mood of the symptoms of this remedy? In what mode, manner and way symptoms of the remedy get worse (aggravated<) or better (ameliorated>) or what is the disposition and temperament (mood) of the symptoms of the remedy.

Now we should understand why in Homoeopathy the mode, the mood, the disposition and the temperament of the symptoms of a remedy, to say more clearly, aggravation and amelioration in the symptoms of a remedy, by different causes, conditions and impressions, are considered so much important? The basic reason for the importance of "MODALITIES" is that the mode and mood of something and changes in it by different impressions and causes indicate its natural and intrinsic qualities. For instance wheat, rather all crops are cultivated in their peculiar weather, condition and atmosphere. It means every seed has an essential natural, intrinsic and basic quality to burst forth and to bud and blossom in its peculiar weather and atmosphere. We can conclusively say here that the qualities of every seed to burst forth, to bud and blossom and to bear fruit in its peculiar weather, condition and atmosphere are its "modalities"--- its essential, natural, intrinsic and basic traits.

In the same manner the mode and the mood, the modalities of the symptoms of a remedy are the remedy's essential natural and intrinsic traits and unless we know and consider the modalities of a remedy we can neither understand it completely nor use it properly. We see that chest complaints of Natrum Sulph are aggravated in warm wet weather and that of Hepar sulph in cold dry weather. Now how can we deny this fact that there is something hidden in Natrum Sulph related to warm wet weather and in Hepar Sulph to cold dry. Medicines have special relation to Modalities peculiar to them. So without considering Modalities that are the essential and intrinsic qualities of medicinal substances, we cannot use them properly.

We see there are certain things soluble in water whereas certain others are insoluble. By burning in the fire certain things are reduced to ashes whereas others become more hard and purified. This is, definitely, because of the essential, natural and intrinsic qualities and properties of things, because of their nature, which mostly differs.

If a medicinal substance produces symptoms by its medicinal effects then, definitely the mode and mood of the symptoms, the modalities of the symptoms, also come from its essential and intrinsic properties. Aggravation and amelioration in the symptoms and all changes in them, brought by different causes and impressions, are hidden and essential constituents of a remedy or disease.

As "modalities" of a remedy denote its intrinsic and essential qualities, in the same manner "modalities" of the symptoms and complaints of a patient identify the intrinsic and integral components of his disease. For instance, pain in throat after cold drinks or painful swelling of throat after swallowing hot foods. Now if swelling, pain, or inflammation in the throat is an aspect of the disease then definitely its aggravation or amelioration by cold or hot drinks is also an essential part and content of the disease because in a state of perfect health a little cold or hot drinks do not harm anyone. One patient has an aggravation in the knee pain by motion and a second patient amelioration by the same. Now if the knee pain is a part of disease why the aggravation or amelioration by motion is not an essential part and indication of the disease?

64 Modalities

In the conventional or other systems of medicine inflammation of throat or pain in the knee, namely, the pathological condition or its material causes are always the basis of the treatment whereas in Homoeopathy merely inflammation of throat or pain in the knee is not all and every thing of the disease. Rather aggravation or amelioration by cold or warm drinks or getting worse or better by motion are also the essential components of the disease. In the same manner some one has headache with sever aggravation in cold air whereas another patient has headache greatly ameliorated in the cold air. So aggravation and amelioration in the symptoms by any action, position, condition and impression is a very firm proof that in spite of the resembling disease conditions in almost every patient there are at least a few internal conditions which are different from others and these internal conditions have a very firm connection with the apparent disease condition. Rather the disease is a collection of its apparent manifestations (symptoms) and hidden parts (modalities). Like other components of symptoms Modalities are also the outcome of disordered vital force. To say more clearly, symptoms are those indications and signs of disease or remedy that appear directly whereas modalities are those hidden and intrinsic indications and signs of the disease or remedy that appear indirectly .... by means of other influences and impressions. Unless all these apparent and hidden signs and indications are found out the picture of either disease or remedy is incomplete and incomprehensible. Therefore, in Homoeopathy, the relationship between symptoms and modalities is always regarded and remedies are selected accordingly. A patient of chest catarrh with aggravation in cold wet weather can be cured by a remedy which has a connection with chest catarrh as well as to the wet weather; rheumatism worse after bathing can be cured by remedies having a relation to rheumatism and bathing as well.

Another reason to keep modalities in view is that most Homoeopathic remedies have marvelous modalities that wonderfully facilitate the selection. If we don't consider modalities of such remedies their correct selection can hardly be made. For instance colic agg. by anger and amel. by pressure and bending double Colocynth. Amel. by walking slowly in cold air, agg. by heat and amel. by consolation Pulsatilla. Agg. by warmth, heat, consolation, at 10 a.m. and amel. by cold Nat-m. Bathing agg., eating and physical exertion amel. Sepia. Bathing, cold and lying agg. and motion amel. Rhus-tox. Motion agg. and pressure amel. Bryonia. Many more such examples can be seen in Homoeopathic Materia Medica.

This is why we should pay a very special attention to the modalities in the study of Materia Medica along with General Symptoms to use remedies correctly according to their apparent and hidden properties.

Modalities are always important as they modify the disease and greatly help us in finding the simillimum. However all modalities don't possess equal importance. Modalities are less or more important according to the concerning symptoms. Modalities related only to particular and less important symptoms are of less importance. Whereas modalities belonging to important general symptoms (mental and physical generals) are the most important. Such modalities play an important role in the selection of a curative remedy.

Sometime beginners take a modality for a symptom and that leads to improper understanding of the totality. If the totality were not precisely understood the selection definitely would be wrong. Kent says,

"I have frequently known young men to mistake a modality for a symptom. This is fatal to a correct result. The symptom is a sensation or condition, and the modality is only a modification. The symptom often becomes peculiar or characteristic through its modality."

(J.T. Kent, Lesser Writings, P. 313)

Important Factors of Modalities

(a) Psychological and Mental Factors

Modalities related to mental and psychological factors are the most important. That is, when Anxiety, Fear, Fright, Grief, Anger, Contradiction, Consolation, Company or Solitude etc., affect symptoms and complaints of patients. These mental and psychological factors greatly help in individualization. In Kent's Repertory psychological and mental factors affecting sensations and complaints have been arranged in such a manner that selection of the remedy has become very easy.

(b) Physical Factors

Physical factors include heat, heat of sun, heat of stove, heat of bed, warm weather dry or wet, cold weather, dry or wet cold weather, cold air, open air, closed rooms etc. In these factors residential places and areas also can be included like environment in schools, colleges, mosques and churches, high and low altitudes, plains and mountains, sea shore etc, because these factors also can bring changes in the symptoms and complaints.

(c) Weather Effects

Changes in weather also cause changes in complaints and symptoms and when used as modalities help in finding appropriate Homoeopathic remedy such as hot or cold weather, rain and snowfalls, thunderstorm, clear or cloudy weather etc.

(d) Time Effects

Many times symptoms and complaints are aggravated or ameliorated at some particular time or in a specific period of life. Day or night, or some peculiar time in 24 hours, morning forenoon or afternoon or at any particular time. Peculiar periods of life such as childhood, youth, old age, puberty, climaxes, periodicity, every 2nd 3rd, 7th or 21st day, moon phases, at new moon, or at full moon and so on. These are also important modalities that help us in arriving at suitable remedy.

(e) Mechanical Effects and Physical Positions

Human actions and activities also play an important role in the aggravation and amelioration of symptoms and complaints. For example aggravation or amelioration by sitting, rising, bending double, lying on the back, or on a side, walking, running, or riding in a carriage and all such conditions and positions also bring changes in symptoms/complaints and help us in completing the picture of disease and finding the exact remedy.

(f) Actions and Functions of Particular Organs

The five senses and different functions and action of other human organs also cause aggravations and ameliorations e.g. noise, odours, touch, appetite, thirst, urination, perspiration, expectoration, menstruation, leucorrhoea, coition, and sleep or sleeplessness etc. These things also bring changes in different states of the disease and the patient and play an important role in shaping the portrait of a totality of symptoms on the basis of which a similar remedy is decided for a patient.

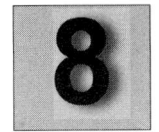

CAUSATIONS

"Causation" means that this remedy can be used for the complaints caused by such and such conditions.

Causes also have been noted down in Materia Medicas and Repertories and require special attention. Causations not only help us in the selection but also in understanding the remedy. In this regard first of all we must understand why certain remedies are considered to be useful for complaints/sufferings arising from or following some cause?

We know every remedy produces its symptoms by means of its natural qualities. Similarly every cause creates symptoms peculiar to it. So according to the law of Similars a remedy can ally the symptoms and complaints following a certain cause only if it has the symptoms following that cause. The remedy suitable for conditions following a cause always has a relation with the symptoms following that cause, not with the cause itself. The reason that Arnica is suitable for mechanical trauma is that it produces symptoms similar to those following a trauma. China and Acid Phos etc. recover the weakness after loss of vital fluids because of having such symptoms in their pathogenesis. Farrington tells us why Hypericum is suitable to the effects of spinal injury,

"HYPERICUM is to be substituted for Arnica when the nerves have been injured along with the other soft parts. Nothing equals Hypericum in case of mashed finger. It relieves the pain and promotes healing. It often follows Arnica in concussion of the spine. Dr. Ludlam of Chicago is very partial to Hypericum in this trouble with the spinal cord, and with good reason, for not only he has relieved some severe cases with it, but the provings show a perfect picture of the results of spinal injury."

(Farrington, Clinical Materia Medica, P. 273)

Another clear explaination of this point is Farrington's recommendation of Veratrum in ailments from fright,

"Veratrum is also to be thought of when after fright, there is great coldness of the body with diarrhoea. GELSEMIUM also has diarrhoea after fright. Under Veratrum, it is associated with coldness and prostration."

(Farrington, Clinical Materia Medica, P. 292)

Nash says about routine of giving Nux-v at start of all cases that have had used allopathic and other drugs,

It would be true if said that Nux vomica will often benefit such cases. The fact is that it will benefit those cases in which the use of such drugs, aromatics, pills, etc. has brought about a condition that simulates the symptoms produced in the provings of Nux vomica, or in cases to which it is homoeopathic and no others. Another fact is that these things often do produce such a condition, and that is one reason why so many physicians are invariably prescribing Nux vomica the first thing, in cases coming from allopathic hands, without even examining the case, but it is unscientific. We have a law of cure and there are cases in which the Nux vomica condition is not present but another more similar remedy must be given. It does not alter the case to say, "Well, I did not know what had been given," for Nux vomica will neither antidote the effects of the drug poison nor cure the disease condition unless it is homoeopathically indicated, especially if given in the dynamic form."

(Nash, Leaders in Homoeopathic Therapeutics, PP. 14-15)

Since every remedy cures only its own symptoms we should always consider its symptoms along with the cause. After a mechanical trauma if there are symptoms of Arnica, Hypericum, Ledum or any other remedy, that must be applied.

Remedies selected merely on the basis of cause sometimes prove to be very effective but at other occasions absolutely fail. This happens when along with cause other symptoms of the remedy are not matched with those of the patient. It is not necessary that there will always be symptoms of Ignatia after a grief. Obviously if there are symptoms of Natrum Mur, Acid Phos, or any other remedy, Ignatia will not benefit. In Kent's repertory under the rubric "Ailments from grief" there is a list of 32 remedies and if a lady is sick after a grief any of these 32 can be her remedy. In the same manner we should not always give China for complaints after the loss of animal fluids. In Kent's repertory under the Rubric "Loss of vital fluids" there are 78 remedies and in every individual case due to this cause we shall need a remedy most similar to the symptoms.

In short the selection of a remedy is always on the basis of symptoms, hence if someone is sick after a specific cause there will be a group of remedies before us, related to that cause, from which we shall choose the most suitable remedy. Therefore we should pay due attention to "Causation" in the study of materia medica to understand and apply medicines correctly.

Sometimes causation plays very important role in the selection because some remedies have a very special connection with the complaints following a specific cause. For example, Nat-s is often suitable for complaints from injuries to head and Arsenic for disordered stomach and vomiting from eating spoiled meat or fish. To understand this point let us read a case of Kent in which he saved his patient by prescribing Nat-s on the basis of causation---injuries to head.

"With the constitutional troubles there are important head symptoms---mental symptoms from injuries of the head. A young man in St. Louis was hurled from a truck in the fire department. He struck on his head. Following this for five or six months he had fits; I do not know what kind of fits he had; some said epilepsy. Some said one thing and some another, and some said he would have to be trephined. He was an

Allopathist, of course, as these firemen all are, for it is hardly ever that you can get one to go outside of Allopathy and try something else. He was a good, well-bred Irishman; so he had to have some good stout physic. Some of his friends prevailed upon him to stay in the country for a while. He did so, but he did not get better; he was irritable; he wanted to die. His wife said she could hardly stand it with him; always wanted to die; did not want to live. His fits drove him to distraction. He did not know when he was going to have one, they were epileptiform in character. Well, in the country he ran across a homeopathic doctor, because he had one of these attacks and the handiest doctor at the time was a Homeopath. That Homeopath told him that he had better come back to St. Louis and place himself under my care. He did so. At that time it had been about six months that he had been having these fits, When he walked into my office he staggered; his eyes were, nearly bloodshot ; he could hardly see, and he wore a shade over his eyes-so much was he distressed about the light such a photophobia. He had constant pain in his head. He had injured himself by falling upon the back of his head and he had with this all the irritability that I have described. There was nothing in his fits that was distinctive of a remedy, and the first thing that came into my head was Arnica; that is what everybody would have thought. Arnica, however, would not have been the best remedy for him. Had I known no other or better remedy, Arnica would have perhaps been the best. As soon as he had finished his description, and I had given the case more thought, I found that Natrum sulphuricum was the best indicated remedy for injuries about the head, and I have been in the habit of giving it. So I gave it in this case. The first dose of Natrum sulphuricum cured this young man. He has never had any pain about the head since. He has never had any mental trouble since, never another fit. That one prescription cleared up the entire case. If you will just remember the chronic effects from injuries upon the skull - not fractures, but simple concussions that have resulted from a considerable shock and injuries without organic affections, then Natrum sulphuricum should be your first remedy. Now, that may not be worth remembering, but when you have relieved as many heads as I have with Natrum sulphuricum you will be glad to have been informed of this circumstance. Ordinarily, Arnica for injuries and the results of injuries, especially the neuralgic pains and the troubles from old scars; but in mental troubles coming on from a jar or a knock on the head or a fall or injury about the head, do not forget this medicine, because if you do many patients may suffer where they might have been cured had you made use of this remedy."

(J.T. Kent, Lectures on Homoeopathic Materia Medica, PP. 789-90)

I also cured a patient of chronic headache by Nat-s. Nearly 17-18 years before he received a severe injury to head. While diving into a pool he struck his head on bottom of the pool and received a severe injury onto vertex. He bled profusely. Since that accident he had headache in occiput and nape of neck which was increasing by the passage of time. He tried all sorts of treatment including homoeopathy but all in vain. Then he came to me. When I looked into the history of the case I found the cause of illness. I also knew that he belonged to a clear-cut sycotic family. There were many rheumatic and asthmatic cases in his family. I gave him a dose of Nat-s 10M which was sufficient for him to get rid of the troublesome long lasting headache.

When I had not dealt with this case I only knew that Nat-s cures the bad effects of injuries to head. But in this case I understood the reason. We know that sycosis weakens the brain. When a sycotic subject receives an injury to head/ brain his tissues of brain do not heal naturally as they should. Since Nat-s is a great and powerful anti-sycotic it overcomes the miasm; the tissues of brain become capable of healing themselves naturally.

Some people suffer from long lasting problems from minor and ordinary causes. For example someone has a small cut by a sharp instrument. His wound does not heal. It suppurates and this suppuration goes on increasing for weeks and months. This is due to a constitutional disordered state in the individual and unless this state is not repaired or yielded the complaint would not be controlled or cured. In these cases a diseased state already exists in the individual and the cause only wakes it up and brings it outward.

Once I was called upon a new born baby who was severely vomiting immediately after birth by caesarean. In the hospital allopathic treatment was applied which failed. They washed the stomach twice but this too could not help. Then I was called and I came to know that the contents of mother's uterus had passed into baby's stomach. I could find no symptoms to prescribe upon except that the baby was restless. Also I did not know and neither I had read about use of Arsenic for vomiting of infants due to contents of uterus passed into stomach; however I knew that Arsenic removes ill effects of bad meat, spoiled fish and ptomaine poison. So I applied it in 30th potency and the baby was quite ok after having 2-3 doses of it. So we see causation serves in practice very much.

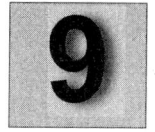

DURATION OF ACTION

"Duration" means how long a remedy can continue its action on an individual.

A medicine, during the provings, continues acting on different provers for different lengths of time and it is due to their differential dispositions and levels of sensitivities. However an average duration of a remedy's action on different provers is considered its "duration of action".

But it does not mean that a remedy necessarily continues acting until the last of its duration time and we cannot repeat it before passing the period of duration or we must repeat it when this period is over. Sensitive patients are influenced by remedies (like other impressions) heavily. It is quite possible that a remedy of 30-40 days duration continues acting on a sensitive patient up to many months or even years. On the other hand a remedy of 60-90 days duration may stop acting within 20-30 days if there is some obstacle due to disease or some counter acting force in the way to recovery. So we would repeat the remedy or take next step before its mentioned duration of action passes.

However from the duration of action we may learn how deeply a remedy may act. Obviously remedies of short duration, from a few hours to a few days, like Aconite or Arnica can help in acute and superficial diseases whereas remedies of long duration like Carbo Veg and Silicia, can cure deep miasmatic maladies.

When a remedy of short duration acts comparatively for a long period, it means the disease is not complicated and the patient will be cured soon and permanently. On the other hand if a remedy of 30 to 40 or 60 to 90 days duration stops acting within a few days it will definitely mean the remedy was not the similimum or the potency was not exact or the pathology was too deep. So it acted superficially and could not start a permanent curative action or it has been antidoted by something or the case is very complicated or incurable. In this way knowledge of duration of action of a remedy helps us managing a case successfully.

10

RELATIONSHIP OF REMEDIES

In relationship of remedies we study effects or influences of other remedies on a particular medicine.

When a remedy has brought some changes, desirable or undesirable, next what remedies we should prefer or avoid. That is when we have to take a turn or next step we would consult relationship of remedies. In relationship of remedies usually the following information is provided.

(i) Complementary remedies.
(ii) Follow well remedies.
(iii) Inimical remedies.
(iv) Antidote remedies

Complementary Remedies

Remedies that revive and promote the curative process started by a previous remedy are called its complementary remedies.

Mostly in chronic cases, and some times in acute ones also, a remedy starts its curative action but before the patient is cured completely the case is stopped and the remedy does not benefit any more in spite of applying it in higher or lower potencies. In such a situation we need a complementary remedy which is often a deeper and more powerful remedy to complete the curative process such as Sulphur after Aconite and Calcarea Carb after Belladonna or Rhus-tox.

A remedy can be complementary to the first one on the basis of its following qualities.

(a) When a remedy has conditions resembling the previous remedy as well as is more deep and powerful such as Sulphur, Kali Carb and Sepia are the complementary remedies to Nux vomica and Ferrum met is complementary to Hamamelis. Farrington says,

"Sulphur is often needed to aid Sepia in chronic cases. The complementary relation lies in the common power of the two drugs to correct abdominal congestion and other vascular irregularities."

(Farrington, Clinical Materia Medica, P. 147)

(b) If a remedy has relieved a miasmatic patient for a while but now the case is stopped then the chief or the most powerful remedy of the concerned miasm can re-establish the curative process such as Sulphur in Psora, Thuja in sycosis and Merc Sol in syphilis.

(c) Or Nosode of the concerned miasm can clear the case or restore the improvement.

We know every remedy acts curatively only on the basis of its symptoms. So when a remedy completes its action but some symptoms have not been cleared, a deep complementary remedy comes to our rescue and often cures the case completely.

Remedies that Follow Well

When a remedy has improved a patient but in the meantime his symptoms have been changed, then we need its Follow Well Remedies.

In chronic and complicated cases mostly a well-selected remedy improves a patient but meanwhile his symptoms change. If the changed image persists for a while, we have to choose a new remedy according to the new totality of the symptoms. So the remedies indicated oftener or acting better after a certain remedy are called its follow well remedies.

It is to be remembered that if a patient needs further treatment, it is not a rule to select a remedy from complementary or follow well remedies. Rather the rule is to retake the case when it has changed positively. Now if the new totality belongs to a follow well or complementary remedy it is good. Otherwise we are bound to follow the symptoms. We do not search the symptoms of follow well and complementary remedies in the patient. Rather we always search a remedy according to the symptoms of the patient.

In regard to making a new selection on a new totality we should also remember that usually changes in the symptoms are a part of the process of cure. The symptoms keep on changing and terminating themselves and the patient is on way towards cure. At this time if we hastily change the remedy it will stop or confuse the case. So if the changed symptoms persist for a considerable length of time (according to the condition or severity of the case) then we can apply aptly a new remedy according to the new totality.

Inimical Remedies

Remedies that are adverse or injurious after a certain remedy are called its "Inimical Remedies"

Contrary to the complementary and follow well remedies there are certain remedies which may confuse or complicate the case if given immediately after certain remedy. Actually any remedy, even an unnecessary dose of the best-fitted remedy can confuse the case. However certain remedies have especially proved, in the experience of experts, to be adverse or inimical to some remedies. If a medicine has made some unfavorable changes in the body its inimical will intensify the suffering or increase the damage already done. Farrington highlights this point as,

"There is this to be remembered, that substances having the same origin generally do not follow each other well. For example, if you have given Ignatia, it is not well to follow it with Nux vomica, and vice versa, because they both contain

Strychnia. Though they have many symptoms in common, they act too much in the same line. Another example may be noted in Glonoin and wine. When Glonoin was proved, it was found to have decided action on the pulse. All the symptoms were aggravated when the provers took wine. Wine produces an excitement very similar to that of Glonoin, but its action seems to be in the same direction, consequently it intensifies the effects of the later."

(Farrington, Clinical Materia Medica, P. 178)

Antidote Remedies

Remedies that can be used to undo or to counteract the effect of certain remedy are called its Antidotes.

The best antidote is the one that covers the troubling symptoms that have come up following the use of a remedy. We can learn how to antidote a medicine by the following description of Farrington,

"The various preparations of Opium enter into the composition of cough-mixtures and soothing syrups used largely in popular practice. Their effects are decidedly pernicious, especially in children. A prominent old-school authority says that the use of soothing-syrup for children is decidedly reprehensible. It stuns their growth, makes them irritable and cross, and interferes sadly with the brain development. Nux vomica is one of the antidotes in cases of injury from anodyne preparations. Still better, perhaps, as an antidote, is Chamomilla, which is suited when opiates have been given for some time, and have produced their secondary effects; the little one is wakeful; slight pains are unbearable. When this condition is present Chamomilla is your remedy, whether the patient is child or adult."

(Farrington, Clinical Materia Medica, PP. 305-6)

We may need to antidote a remedy in the following situations.

(a) When a medicine produces some troubling symptoms and its action needs to be modified. Farrington says,

"Then again there are drugs which antidote each other. You may have made a mistake. Your patient may be too susceptible to the action of the remedy, and you require to modify its action. It was only yesterday that I prescribed Nux vomica for a cold. It relived the patient of his cold, but he became almost crazy with headache. He had an axcess of Nux vomica, so I gave him Coffea, and in minutes his head was better. This was done simply by modifying the effects of Nux vomica, not by suppressing the symptoms."

(Farrington, Clinical Materia Medica, P. 7)

(b) When a remedy changes symptoms in the wrong direction. For instance there starts some heart trouble after joints pains having been relieved. It means the remedy applied caused a metastasis of the disease from less important organs towards more important organs.

(c) When in a case of critical pathologies there starts a threatening aggravation. (In this situation one or a few doses of the same remedy in smaller potency (12c, 30c) subside the undesirable aggravation and improvement starts without antidoting the remedy).

(d) When in a case of an extremely weak or incurable patient the similar remedy affects the vital force as a harmful medicinal substance instead of a curative agent. To say more clearly the vital force is too weak to react and the medicine starts producing its symptoms instead of eradicating the disease symptoms.

Though in the earlier literature of Homoeopathy it has been taught to antidote the first remedy in the conditions mentioned above, yet present renowned teachers, like George Vithoulkas, advise not to antidote a homoeopathic remedy with another homoeopathic one. This is because the antidotal remedy produces new complications and ambiguities along with antidoting the effects of the first remedy. Probably the difference between these old and new viewpoints is because in the old times such high potencies were not commonly used that we use today. If a remedy in a low potency had produced undesirable effects it was antidoted with another remedy in the low potency without any further complications. But now, as we know, there are in use very high potencies of Homoeopathic remedies and if a deep acting remedy starts producing undesirable changes and we apply an antidote, possibly it will not be able to antidote the first remedy fully, or before antidoting the first the second will produce its own ill effects and complications will take place. In this situation the first strategy sould be, if the condition allows, let some time pass and exhaust the medicine itself. If severity or rapid development of the symptoms does not allow proper wait then we would have to antidote the first applied medicine.

"When the selected remedy acts not in accordance with Herings' law of cure, and when the peripheral symptoms improve but the mind and other life-sustaining organs are threatened, it needs to be antidoted. It can be antidoted by clinically verified and mentioned antidotes, e.g. Arsenicum album can be antidoted by Camphora, Nux vomica, Hepar Sulfuris or Graphites. Another method to antidote would be to assess the case again and take the whole picture into account, the original and the new symptoms of the patient and choose the remedy which covers the totality. This works in my experience often wonders. Smelling of Camphor or drinking large quantities of herb teas or coffee etc. can also bring down the intensity of the unwanted symptoms but may not always suffice to affect the disturbed dynamic plane."

(Paragraph added by Dr. Mohinder Singh Jus, SHI Switzerland)

These hints were about the common uses of antidotes. Now, here, I give a hint about a special use of them. We know a remedy antidotes another one on the basis of similar symptoms. The more similar symptoms a remedy has the more suitable antidote it is. So if a remedy fails on a patient, we can choose second remedy for him from the list of its antidotes because antidotes also have resembling symptoms and conditions. If we succeed in finding the appropriate remedy from the list of antidotes it will not only start its positive action but also antidote the undesired effects of the first one if there were any. Hahnemann says in aphorism 166,

"...and the bad effects resulting from it, when they do occur, are diminished whenever a subsequent medicine, of more accurate resemblance, can be selected"

(Hahnemann, Organon, P. 224)

COMPARISON WITH RESEMBLINNG REMEDIES

H.C. Allen says in the preface to his "Keynotes of Leading remedies",

"The life work of the student of the homoeopathic Materia Medica is one of constant comparison and differentiation. He must compare the pathogenesis of a remedy with recorded anamnesis of the patient; he must differentiate the apparently similar symptoms of two or more medicinal agents in order to select the similimum."

(H.C. Allen, Keytones, P.5)

Usually under every remedy there is a note, "Compare:" (it to these remedies). It means these remedies also have symptoms and conditions similar to the remedy under study and if you are going to apply it to a patient have a look at or ponder over these remedies also. This comparative study of remedies, before making a selection, is very important because where there is resemblance in the symptoms of some remedies there is some difference also and that difference is our guide in making a selection. If we look at all the comparable remedies before making a selection the most appropriate remedy certainly will come before us. If one cannot differentiate remedies from one another one would not be able to decide on the best suitable one. Farrington says,

"You go into a field and you see two or three hundred cattle. They all look alike to you, yet the man in charge of them knows each one. How does he know them? He knows them by certain distinctions which he has learned by familiarity with them. So can you know one drug from another by studying their points of difference. Drugs impinge in their resemblances, and separate in their differences. Thus we have another form of study, comparison of drugs. That is just as necessary to successful practice as is the first step, the analysis of the drugs."

(Farrington, Clinical Materia Medica, P. 7)

We can compare remedies with the help of comparable remedies given under every remedy in the Materia Medica. Also there are special comparative Materia Medicas from which H.A. Robert's "The Study of Remedies by Comparison" and A. Gaskin's "Comparative Study on Kent's Materia Medica" are easy and very useful. There are two more classics "Comparative Materia Medica" by Gross and "Comparative Materia Medica by Farrington".

STUDY OF CURED CASES

J.T. Kent says about understanding and retaining Materia Medica,

" To be constantly at hand, it must be constantly and correctly used".

(J.T. Kent, Lectures on Homoeopathic Materia Medica, P. 12)

When we select a remedy according to the symptoms and the patient is cured it means we have sketched a clear and recognizable picture of the remedy and its patient in our mind. Next time we will easily recognize these patients. But it is difficult rather impossible for a student or beginner of Homeopathy to have many patients of a remedy and observe its effects on them. So the solution to this problem is to study the cured cases of a remedy as many as possible. When we read that certain remedy was selected for such a patient on the basis of these symptoms along with these conditions and he was cured, a precise and practical picture of the remedy sets in our mind that cannot be achieved by merely reading the symptomatology in the Materia Medica.

Moreover when we study many different cases cured by a remedy, different aspects of the remedy appear before us and we become aware of its full use in different conditions and diseases. It is my personal experience that after the study of cured cases of certain remedies their selection was always easy and successful in my practice.

To study the cured cases by renowned Homoeopaths Gunavante's "Amazing Power of Homoeopathy" is a very useful book. In the first section of the book he has presented

201 cases of renowned and genius Homoeopaths cured by different remedies in the form of exercise. And in second section the symptoms extracted from the case and the selected remedy of every case has been mentioned as solution of the exercise. The more cured cases of a remedy do we study the more we are well acquainted with its use in different conditions and diseases. Gunavante says,

"Readers are advised to study each of the following cases, as if it is presented to them for treatment – finding the curative remedy – by referring to the Repertory as well as the Materia Medica. Thorough search for the remedy in each case, if need be taking a day or two for it, will greatly enhance your knowledge of the 'genius' or 'essence' of the various remedies in the materia medica and will help you to become a more efficient, accurate and speedy prescriber than you have ever been."

(Gunavante, Amazing Power of Homoeopathy, P. 1)

N.M. Chudhuri's "A Study on Materia Medica" is a wonderful book in this respect. After elaborating a remedy he gives some cases cured by it that makes the reader understand the remedy in a very practical way. Another book is "Testimoy of Clinic" by E.B. Nash.

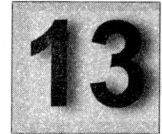

THE APPROPRIATE POTENCY

Some Materia Medicas, like Boericke's "Pocket Manual" and K.N. Mathur's "Systematic Materia Medica" indicate the effective potencies of remedies. Although some particular potencies of certain remedies have been mentioned to be comparatively more effective, yet selection of potency depends on constitution of the patient and condition or stage of the disease rather than the origin of the remedy. In Kent's words,

"The various potencies are all more or less related to individuals and it is the individual that we should study".

(J.T. Kent, Lesser Writings, P. 347)

Thus the selection of potency becomes a subject directly related to philosophy, rather than Materia Medica. However, homeopathic philosophy books that shed some light on this topic are very rare and the information provided in them also seems varying. Probably this is the reason that most students are not trained well or they are absolutely unaware of this indispensable part of Homoeopathic prescribing. Some beginners habitually use low potencies ranging from "Q" (mother tincture) to 30th or 200th being the later their highest. Others apply indiscriminately high potencies ranging from 30th or 200th to CM or DM and MM if available. This group starts nearly every case from 200, 1M or 10M and both groups are often seen criticizing each other.

If we realistically observe and compare the results achieved by both the low and the high potencies, we witness marvelous cures produced by all of them. We also see that a certain potency, be it low or high, fails in a case while some other potency cures the case completely. So instead of adopting an arbitrary mode for selection of potency we should understand the factors which correspond to the different effects of different potencies.

Actually a perfect similar remedy produces some effects but the action of an improper potency may be greatly less or more than needed for a rapid, gentle and permanent cure. If the potency is too low for the patient's constitution and condition of the disease it will not produce a complete cure or possibly any noticeable change. Also frequent repetition of a medicine in too low a potency may be dangerous in some cases. On the other hand a very high potency may cause a powerful unnecessary aggravation even threatening for the life of the patient.

We can find basic guidelines on the selection of potency in some of Kent's articles in his "Lesser Writings". In addition Stuart Close has written a full chapter on Homoeopathic posology in "The Genius of Homoeopathy". Stuart Close throws light on different conditions that demand different potencies; elaborates the involving factors encompassing all aspects along with presenting example cases. George Vithoulkas also gives very useful hints in "The Science of Homoeopathy. Gunavante in his "Introduction to Homoeopathic Prescribing" has also provided very helpful information presenting quotes from J.T.Kent, H.A.Roberts, Carol Dunham, Borland, F.Hubbard, Stuart Close and many other experts. Dr. Mohinder Singh Jus also gives in "The Journey of a Disease" some useful points especially highlighting importance of lower potencies. A summary of the information contained in the mentioned sources is presented here, in original words, so that the reader may conceive a clear and broad concept of the subject in a concise way.

START AND GRADUAL DEVELOPMENT OF THE POTENCY SYSTEM

Hahnemann's final views and practice in regard to the dose were arrived at gradually, through long years of careful experiment and observation; at first even for some time after the promulgation of the law of similars and the method of practice based upon it, he used medicines in material doses and in the usual form. His discovery of the principle of potentiation came about gradually as he experimented in the reduction of his doses, in order, to arrive at a point where severe aggravations would not occur. Gradually, by experience, he learned that the latent powers of drugs were released or developed by trituration, dilution and succussion. Thus he arrived at his final conclusion that the proper dose is always the least possible dose which will affect a cure.

(Stuart Close, The Genius of Homoeopathy, PP. 189-90)

"When he witnessed the fearful aggravations from crude doses of the "similar" remedies, he started the procedure of "reducing" the dose, and the small dose was first called "dilution". To this process of dilution, Hahnemann had added another far reaching condition, viz., at firs two, but later ten forceful strokes, called succussion, given to the dilution at each stage.

(Gunavante, Introduction to Homoeopathic Prescribing, P. 126)

"In the fifth edition of the Organon Hahnemann laid down clear instructions for making potencies on the centesimal scale. According to this method, one drop of the strong tincture of a soluble drug is put in a small bottle with ninety-nine drops of alcohol, and this is vigorously succussed. This becomes the first centesimal potency. Subsequent potencies are prepared in the same way — always one drop of the preceding potency in ninety-nine drops of attenuating medium, to form the next higher potency".

"With the insoluble substances, such as gold, silica, carbon, Lycopodium, etc., Hahnemann made first potencies by trituration (one part of the substance in ninety-nine parts of sugar of milk, triturated in an agate mortar for a couple of hours). One part of its first centesimal trituration is again ground up with ninety-nine parts of sugar of milk for the same period, to make a second centesimal potency, and a third potency is made in the same way. That gives the substance, as one in a million. And he shows that after these three triturations all substances become soluble in alcohol or water and potencies can now be run up in the usual way".

(Gunavante, Introduction to Homoeopathic Prescribing, PP.126-27)

Posology, and the related subject of Potentiation were the subjects of so much misunderstanding, discussion and controversy in the early days of homeopathy that the profession, after being divided into two opposing camps, grew tired of the subject. It came to be regarded as a kind of "Gordian Knot" to be cut by each individual as best he could with instruments at his disposal. Hahnemann himself at one time, almost in despair of ever being able to bring his followers to an agreement on the subject, cut the knot by proposing to treat all cases with the thirtieth potency. Following this suggestion others tacitly adopted a dosage confined to one, or a very limited range of potencies. The materialistically minded restricted themselves to the crude tinctures and triturations, or the very low dilutions, ranging from 1x to 6x. Others ranged from the third to the thirtieth potencies, while another class of metaphysical tendency used only the very high potencies, ranging from the two hundredth to the millionth, each according to his personal predilection.

(Stuart Close, The Genius of Homoeopathy, PP. 183-84)

In the early years homoeopathic physicians used to make the potencies by their own hand in all ranges, such as 30, 200, 500, 2,000, 48M and so on. There was no regular scale of potencies.

It goes to the credit of Dr, J.T.Kent that he brought order out of chaos.

(Gunavante, Introduction to Homoeopathic Prescribing, P. 127)

After a long observation in the range of potencies, going up and down, I have settled upon the octaves in the series of degrees as —30th, 200th, 1M, 10M, 50M, CM, DM and MM. Many of my patients' records indicate that the patient has steadily improved after each potency, to the highest, with symptoms becoming fainter, and he himself growing stronger, mentally and physically.

(J.T. Kent, Lesser Writings, P. 359)

I once used potencies that ranged nearer to each other, but repeatedly found that the degrees must be far enough apart to represent an octave, or failure followed. I observed that after the good action of a 200th, after waiting until it was no longer active, although I gave the 300, 500, and 800, the 1M acted much more strongly; and the 300 or 500 generally failed.

(J.T. Kent, Lesser Writings, P. 358)

Many times I used to give first a CM, but found that when going lower the action was seldom so strong as when climbing upward. Again, I often observed sharp aggravation when beginning the CM, but seldom observed aggravation when beginning low in relation to the sensitiveness of my patient's nature.

(J.T. Kent, Lesser Writings, P. 359)

As a rule, two doses (sometimes three) in the same plane give the best results. It has become almost routine, as the records indicate that the third dose in the same potency gives no effect.

(J.T. Kent, Lesser Writings, PP. 351-52)

As everyone is aware, the potencies now available are all made in these series. In our discussion, "low" potencies would mean Mother Tincture (Q) to 12c: "medium would mean 30c. and 200c. : and high from 1M upwards (10M, 50M), the "highest" being CM, DM, MM, etc.

(Gunavante, Introduction to Homoeopathic Prescribing, P. 127)

SCALES OF HOMOEOPATHIC POTENCIES

Decimal Scale

The decimal scale is based on dilution of 1/10. The first 1x potency is 1/10 dilution. The dilution (1/10 X 1/10= 1/100) is called 2x potency. (And so on)

Centesimal Scale

The centesimal scale is the most commonly used in homoeopathy. It is based upon serial dilutions of 1/100. Each centesimal potency, therefore, is equivalent in dilution to two decimal potencies. A 30c potency is the same as a 60x, considering only the amount of dilution.

(Vithoulkas, The Science of Homoeopathy, P. 164)

Fifty-Millesimal Scale

About the year 1840, roughly 4 years before his death Hahnemann modified the preparation of potencies to the 50 millesimal scale obviously after satisfying himself through experiment with their greater advantages. He incorporated instruction about the method of making them in paragraph 270 of the revised Sixth edition of the Organon. However, as the edition remained with his widow and thereafter went into the hands of her daughter, it became available to the homoeopathic world only in 1921, about 80 years late, through efforts of William Boericke. Meanwhile, during the long interregnum, Dr, Hering, Kent, E.E.Case, C.M.Boger, Adolph Lippe, Nash and many other pioneers achieved marvelous results form the centesimal scale of potencies. As working of these 50 millesimals potencies is quite different and because of paucity of wide experience with them even now a majority of homoeopaths all over the world are using the centesimal scale of potencies. In India Dr. Ramanlal P. Patel has written My Experiments with 50 Millesimal Scale of Potency. It is claimed on their behalf that 50 Millesimal are (i) less liable to produce medicinal aggravations even in highly sensitive patients and (ii) they can be repeated every day in acute as well as in chronic disease.

(Gunavante, Introduction to Homoeopathic Prescribing, P. 128)

Another useful book on this Hahnemann's finally advised scale is "50 Millesimal Potency in Theory and Practice" by Harimohan Choudhury. In this book he has provided a complete knowledge about this scale, describing its history, theory, mode of preparation and application with its advantages in the practice.

The mode of preparation is given below in brief since the details can be had from the Organon (sixth) itself:

We should prepare three successive triturations (i.e. 1st, 2nd and 3rd trituration) from the original substance (or mother substance). The ratio of each will be 1/100. Take on one grain from 3rd trituration and dissolve it (by necessary shaking) in 500 drops (100 drops of alcohol and 400 drops of distilled water). This is the 4th stratum. We call this stage, 'The Mother Potency' of the new method. The ratio is 1/500.

One drop from this 4th stage is to be mixed with 100 drops of alcohol. This is to be succussed 100 times. This is the 1st potency (or M/1, or 0/1 or LM/1, etc.) of the new method. Proportion is 1/50,000.

With one drop of this 1st potency (i.e. LM/1) 500 globules (of which 100 weigh 1gr, i.e. No 10 globules) are to be soaked. Then put one such medicated globule in a vial and put in it one drop of distilled water for its dissolution. Then put 100 drops of alcohol in the vial and succuss it 100 times. This is the

2nd potency (i.e. LM/2) of the new method. The ratio of it is 1/50,000 or more.

In this way the dynamization may be raised from LM/3 to LM/30 or as needed.

(Harimohan, 50Millesimal Potency in Theory and Practice, PP. 8-9)

NECESSITY AND ADVANTAGE OF MAXIMUM RANGE OF POTENCIES

The physician who knows how to use the various potencies has ten times the advantage of the one that always uses one potency, no matter what the potency is.

(J.T. Kent, Lesser Writings, P. 207)

Individualization in regard to potencies as in other branches of homoeopathic work, furnishes us with an additional element of accuracy and success, enabling us to reach certain cases that we otherwise could not reach.

(J.T. Kent, Lesser Writings, P. 347)

Several times I have seen patients on repeated doses of a right remedy in a low potency make no improvement, simply because their susceptibility to that potency— not to that remedy by any means— had been exhausted. I have taken such patients and without changing the remedy but simply the potency got a curative result.

(J.T. Kent, Lesser Writings, P. 348)

It is not an uncommon recital in the record that the patient continues to improve on each potency for three or four months. Any physician who learns the use of these degrees in chronic diseases possesses the untold advantages over the physician with his one potency.

(J.T. Kent, Lesser Writings, PP. 359-60)

Many chronic sicknesses are cured by keeping the patient under the influence of the one indicated remedy for two or more years. But this cannot be done, with continuous curative action, unless the doctrine of series in degrees is fully understood and used.

(J.T. Kent, Lesser Writings, P. 357)

The indiscriminate use of any one potency is very likely to bring reproach upon our art.

(J.T. Kent, Lesser Writings, P. 347)

The selection of the remedy can hardly be said to be finished until the potency and dosage have been decided upon. These three factors, remedy, potency and dosage, are necessarily involved in the operation of prescribing. Not one of them is a matter of indifference and not one of them can be disregarded.

(Stuart Close, The Genius of Homoeopathy, P. 202)

Each man should be competent, willing and ready to use any potency or preparation of the remedy indicated in a given case, without prejudice. If he confines himself to one or two potencies, be they low, medium, or high, he is limiting his own usefulness and depriving his patients of valuable means of relief and cure.

(Stuart Close, The Genius of Homoeopathy, P. 184)

Practitioners who publicly boast of their liberality on this subject, will too often be found, on more intimate acquaintance, to practice an obstinate exclusivism in the use of some particular potency, generally a very low or a very high one; and to harshly criticize those who differ with them. This is unfortunate, because such practitioners undoubtedly deprive themselves and their patients of many agents of cure which are easily within their reach.

(Stuart Close, The Genius of Homoeopathy, P. 191)

REQUIRED RANGE OF POTENCIES AS SUGGESTED BY EXPERTS

Every physician should have at command the 30th, 200th, 1M, 10M, 50M, CM, DM and MM potencies, made carefully on the centesimal scale.

(J.T. Kent, Lesser Writings, P. 207)

The great bulk of the work of the profession, however, is done with lower and medium potencies and these, if accurately prescribed and wisely managed, will give satisfactory results in great majority of cases. The third, sixth, twelfth, and thirtieth potencies with a set of the two hundredth to "top of with" gives a general working range. When the young practitioner can afford to add to these a set of BOERICKE & TAFEL'S hand made five hundredths and one thousandths, he will be well equipped indeed. The rest is "velvet;" but if any body should offer him a set of Finke's, Swan's or Skinner's fifty thousandths and one hundred thousandths, he should not let his modesty nor his prejudices prevent him from accepting and trying them. Hundreds of practitioners, including the writer, have used them with great satisfaction.

(Stuart Close, The Genius of Homoeopathy, P. 191)

An old man with an enlarged prostate who is so weakened that he spends most of his time in bed would be given a 12x (or sometimes even a 6x) potency only daily.

The homoeopathic information leads to a very clear picture of Pulsatilla, and your observation of the patient confirms this expression. In such a case, you could easily prescribe Pulsatilla 50M or even CM with confidence.

(Vithoulkas, The Science of Homoeopathy, PP. 215-16)

GENERAL GUIDELINES FOR DIFFERENT DEGREES OF POTENCIES

There is a wonderful latitude between the tinctures and the CMs and in my judgment the selection of the best potency is a matter of experience and observation and not as yet a matter of law.
(J.T. Kent, Lesser Writings, P. 347)

Once a remedy is selected, the next decision facing the prescriber is the choice of potency. For this, there are no set rules, and experience and observation play a very large role. In this section, some general guidelines will be presented, but it must be fully understood that they are not designed to be adopted as "rules".
(Vithoulkas, The Science of Homoeopathy, P. 213)

High Potencies

In acute diseases 1M and 10M are the most useful.

From 10M to the MM are all useful for all ordinary chronic diseases in persons not so sensitive.

In persons suffering from chronic sickness and not so sensitive, the 10M may first be used, and continued without change so long as improvement lasts; then the 50M will act precisely in the same manner, and should be used so long as the patient makes progress toward health; then the CM may be used in the same manner, and the DM and MM in succession. By this use of the series of potencies in a given case, the patient can be held under the influence of the similimum, or a given remedy, until cured.
(J.T. Kent, Lesser Writings, P. 207)

The more similar the remedy, the more clearly and positively the symptoms of a patient take on the peculiar and characteristic form of the remedy, the greater the susceptibility to that remedy, and the higher the potency required.

(Stuart Close, The Genius of Homoeopathy, P. 192)

Generally speaking, susceptibility is greatest in children and young, vigorous persons, and diminishes with age. Children are particularly sensitive during development, and the most sensitive organs are those which are being developed. Therefore the medicines which have a peculiar affinity for those organs should be given in the medium or higher potencies.

The higher potencies are best adopted to sensitive persons of the nervous, sanguine or choleric temperament; to intelligent, intellectual persons, quick to act and react; to zealous and impulsive persons.

(Stuart Close, The Genius of Homoeopathy, P. 194)

If the potency is too high its action may be too deep and far reaching, and the reaction too great for the weakened vital power to carry on. Such remedies as Sulphur, Calc-c, Mercurius, Arsenic and Phosphorus, given in the 50M or CM potencies, have sometimes hastened tubercular or tertiary syphilis cases into the grave. In the beginning of treatment of such suspicious or possibly incurable cases it is better to use medium potencies, like the 30th or 200th and go higher gradually, if necessary, as treatment progresses and the patient improves.

(Stuart Close, The Genius of Homoeopathy, P. 207)

When the symptoms of a case clearly indicate one remedy, whose characteristic symptoms correspond closely to the characteristic symptoms of the case, we give high potencies— thirtieth, two hundredth, thousandth, or higher according to the prescriber's degree of confidence and the contents of his medicine case.

(Stuart Close, with reference to Jahr, The Genius of Homoeopathy, PP. 183-84)

If a case seems relatively curable and free of physical pathology, higher initial potencies may be tried, ranging from

30 to CM. The primary guiding principle here is the degree of certainty which the homoeopath has about the remedy. If the medicine seems very obvious and covers the case very well, a very high potency may be given to a person with a curable system. If the remedy is not so clear, it is better to begin with a potency closer to 30.

(Vithoulkas, The Science of Homoeopathy, P. 215)

In children with acute ailments (because their defensive mechanisms are quite strong), it is best not to give potencies lower than 200; thus 200 to CM potencies can be given, depending upon certainty of the medicine for acute ailments

(Vithoulkas, The Science of Homoeopathy, P. 217)

An M.D with a few years' experience in homoeopathy attempted to treat a child suffering from severe mental disorders. The patient had received approximately fifteen remedies, some of which had partial actions and others of which had no action. The case was sent to me and the case taken during the initial interview showed clearly Veratrum Album, which had been given only as the tenth prescription amidst a variety of others. Based upon this initial interview, Veratrum Album 50M (it is best to go high potencies if possible in such cases) was given again with instructions to wait after that for a full three months in order to fully evaluate direction of the remedy.

(Vithoulkas, The Science of Homoeopathy, PP. 251-52)

Medium Potencies

From 30th to 10M will be found those curative powers most useful in very sensitive women and children.

In sensitive women and children, it is well to give the 30th or 200th at first, permitting the patient to improve in a general way, after which the 1M may be used in similar manner. After improvement with that ceases, the 10M may be required.

(J.T. Kent, Lesser Writings, P. 207)

Some patients are very sensitive to the highest potencies and are cured mildly and permanently by the use of 200th or 1000th. There are other individuals who are torn to pieces by the use of the highest potencies.

Patients who have heart disease, or who are suffering from phthisis are apt to have their sufferings increased and the end hastened by the higher potencies; they do better under 30th or 200th.

(J.T. Kent, Lesser Writings, P. 347)

If you strike too high she is not sensitive, it is not sufficient. Keep to the mild potency so long as it works. It is not well to jump too many degrees. From the crude to 10M there is a range of degrees in ordinary person.

(J.T. Kent, Lesser Writings, P. 350)

Sulphur, like silica, is a dangerous medicine to give where there is structural disease in organs that are vital, especially the lungs. Sulphur will often heal old fistulous pipes and turn old abscesses into a normal state, so that healthy pus will follow, when it is indicated by the symptoms. It will open abscesses that are very slow, doing nothing, it will reduce inflamed glands that are indurated and about to suppurate, when the symptoms agree. But it is a dangerous medicine to administer in advanced cases of phthisis, and, if given, it should not be prescribed in the highest potencies. If there are symptoms that are very painful, and you think that Sulphur must be administered, go to the 30th or 200th potency".

(J.T. Kent, Lectures on Materia Medica, P. 958)

A single dose of the appropriate nosode (In a case, which is not at all susceptible to the indicated remedy) in a moderately high potency, will sometimes clear up the case by brining symptoms into view which will make it possible to select the remedy required to carry on the case.

(Stuart Close, The Genius of Homoeopathy, P. 202)

A correctly chosen remedy given in too low or sometimes too high a potency, or in too many doses, may cause an aggravation of the existing symptoms as to endanger the life of the patient; especially if the patient be a child or a sensitive person and if a vital organ, like the brain or lung be affected. Belladonna in the third or sixth potency, given in too frequent doses in a case of meningitis, for example, may cause death from over-action; whereas the thirtieth or two hundredth potency given in single dose or in doses repeated only until some change of symptoms is noticed, will speedily cure. Phosphorus 3rd or 6th in pneumonia under similar circumstances may rapidly cause death. The low potencies of deeply acting medicines are dangerous in such cases in proportion to their similarity to the symptoms.

(Stuart Close, *The Genius of Homoeopathy*, P. 206)

Oversensitive patients present a unique problem for potency selection. There are patients who are excessively "nervous" reactive to all physical and emotional stimuli, usually lean and quick in their movements, restless, sensitive to odors and noise and light, and frequently suffering strongly from exposure to chemicals in the environment or food. Such people are very reactive both to low potencies (on physical level) and high potencies (on electrodynamic level). Consequently, it is better to restrict initial prescriptions to 30 or 200 in such patients; depending upon their reaction, later potencies might go higher or lower. But initially at least, 30 or 200 are the best selections for oversensitive patients

(Vithoulkas, *The Science of Homoeopathy*, P. 215)

On the other hand, another young lady comes to you with similar complaint, but you cannot decide weather she needs Pulsatilla or Sulphur. You finally decide upon Pulsatilla after many hours of careful study; in this instance, you would tend to give only a 30 or 200 for the initial prescription because of the lack of clarity.

In still another case with a skin eruption, you may see clearly that Pulsatilla is indicated. Yet the patient reports that she was able to keep her skin eruption under control by using cortisone ointment "only" twice a week. Further you observe that there are other weaknesses of the organism—a weak vitality, the patient is easily tired, easily affected by chemicals in the environment. In this type of case you would not give a potency higher than 200; otherwise you may witness an unnecessary prolonged aggravation.

(Vithoulkas, *The Science of Homoeopathy*, PP. 216-17)

If the patient is elderly, chronically weakened, or even if severely weakened by the acute ailment (for example, if it has developed into a severe pneumonia), a 200 potency would be preferable for the initial prescription, even if the remedy is quite obvious.

(Vithoulkas, *The Science of Homoeopathy*, P. 217)

Low Potencies

Sometimes very sensitive patients will do well on a high potency if they have been prepared for it by the use of a lower one.

(J.T. Kent, *Lesser Writings*, P. 347)

I have seen Sulphur and Phosphorus act so strongly that I have regretted it. In lung cases, consider whether she has lung space enough to make recovery probable. If she can bear it, give it in low potency; but do not give it if there is not lung space enough to warrant it.

(J.T. Kent, *Lesser Writings*, P. 351)

Where the symptoms are not clearly developed and there is an absence or scarcity of characteristic features; or where two or three remedies seem about equally indicated, susceptibility and reaction may be regarded as low. We give, therefore, the remedy which seems most similar, in a low (third to twelfth) potency.

(Stuart Close, with reference to Jahr, The Genius of Homoeopathy, P. 193)

Lower potencies and larger and frequent doses correspond better to torpid and phlegmatic individuals, dull of comprehension and slow to act; to coarse fibered, sluggish individuals of gross habits; to those who possess great muscular power but who require a powerful stimulus to excite them. Such persons can take with seeming impunity large amounts of stimulants like whisky, and show little effect from them. When ill they often require low potencies, or even sometimes material doses.

(Stuart Close, The Genius of Homoeopathy, P. 194)

If the grade of the disease is low, and the power of reaction low, the remedy must be given low. Thus we find, in such cases, that the symptoms of the patient are usually of a low order; common, pathological symptoms; organ symptoms; gross terminal symptoms; symptoms that correspond to the effects of crude drugs in massive toxic doses. The finer shadings of symptoms belonging to acute conditions, in vigorous sensitive patients, do not appear. Potentiated medicines will not act. The case has passed beyond that stage, and finer symptoms with it. Yet the symptoms remain and the almost hopeless conditions they represent, are still within the scope of the homoeopathic law; and they sometimes yield to its power, when the related law of posology is rightly understood and applied.

(Stuart Close, The Genius of Homoeopathy, P. 195)

People who are accustomed to long and severe labour out-of-doors, who sleep little and whose food is coarse, are less susceptible. Persons exposed to continual influence of drugs, such as tobacco workers and dealers; distillers and brewers and all connected with the liquor and tobacco trade; druggist, perfumers, chemical workers, etc. often possess little susceptibility to medicines and usually require low potencies in the illnesses.

(Stuart Close, The Genius of Homoeopathy, P. 199)

The seat, character and intensity of the disease has some bearing upon the question of the dose. Certain malignant and rapidly fatal diseases, like cholera, may require material doses or low potencies of the indicated drug.

(Stuart Close, The Genius of Homoeopathy, P. 200)

Occasionally a case will be met which is not at all susceptible to the indicated remedy. Hahnemann has recommended in such cases, the administration of Opium, in one of the lowest potencies, every eight or twelve hours until some signs of reaction are perceptible. By this, he says, the susceptibility is increased and the new symptoms of the diseases are brought to light. Carbo-veg, Laurocerasus, Sulphur and Thuja are other remedies suited to such conditions. They sometimes serve to arouse the organism to reaction so that indicated remedies will act.

(Stuart Close, The Genius of Homoeopathy, PP. 201-2)

There are certain types of cases in which relatively low potencies should be used— at least initially. Patients who have weak constitutions, old people, or very hypersensitive people should initially be given potencies ranging, roughly, from 12x to 200. The reason for this is that higher potencies can over stimulate the weakened defense mechanism, resulting in unnecessary powerful aggravations.

(Vithoulkas, The Science of Homoeopathy, P. 214)

Children who are suffering from severe problems should generally be given low potencies. An infant with severe eczema or psoriasis is likely to have severe aggravation if given a high potency. Consequently, such cases might be given just a few doses (say daily) of a 12x, or just one dose of a 30 or 200.

Generally, cases with known malignancy should not initially be given potencies above 200. If a case is merely suspected to have a malignant or premalignant condition, the initial prescription should not be higher than 1M. Again such potency restriction is in order to avoid unnecessary powerful physical aggravations, which require considerable experience to manage.

(Vithoulkas, The Science of Homoeopathy, P. 215)

* * *

CONCLUSION

Upon reading superficially, the descriptions of Kent, Stuart Close, George Vithoulkas and other experts regarding the lowest and the highest potencies seem varying. Kent suggests 30 as the lowest. Vithoulkas does not go lower than 6x where as Stuart Close advises to apply the lowest preparations (3x, Q, even material doses) if necessary. This may be confusing for a student. But we may easily clear the confusion if we ponder over these descriptions a bit deeper. When we study the conditions for which these suggestions have been made, we may easily conclude that these are not varying suggestions; rather these are suggestions made for different conditions. Kent has suggested 30 as the lowest for common cases as we come across in our routine practice. Although he had a metaphysical tendency and was inclined to higher potencies yet he did not strictly forbid us to use potencies lower than 30. How can he (a wise prescriber) restrain us from using a low potency when it is necessary? He says,

"There is a wonderful latitude between the tinctures and the CMs and in my judgment the selection of the best potency is a matter of experience and observation and not as yet a matter of law."

(J.T. Kent, Lesser Writings, P. 347)

From the crude to 10M there is a range of degrees in ordinary person.

(J.T. Kent, Lesser Writings, P. 350)

These statements of Kent clearly open before us all ways to utilize the maximum range of potencies. If we agree that there are some cases which need 30 instead of 10M or 1M, why there may not be some others which would be in need of 12x, 6x or lower.

Vithoulkas suggests 12x or 6x for severe pathological cases, or that are suspected to have an intense aggravation from higher potencies. Whereas Stuart Close advises not to miss the advantage of the lowest potencies in cases which do not respond to highly potentiated forms of medicines. He says,

"In certain terminal conditions the power of the organism to react, even to indicated homoeopathic remedy, may become so low that only material doses can arouse it. A common example of this is seen in certain terminal conditions of valvular heart disease, where Digitalis is the indicated remedy, but no effect is produced by any potency."

(Stuart Close, The Genius of Homoeopathy, P. 194)

To justify his statement Stuart Close describes a case from his practice in which Digitalis had failed in all potencies. But an allopathic physician applied it in material doses and the case was cured. Further, he says that all occasional successes of allopathic physicians in such cases are essentially, although crudely, homoeopathic. Allopathic physicians do, in such cases what the homoeopathic physician should have discernment and common sense to do; — namely, give the drug that is really homoeopathic to the case, but give it in the stronger doses required at that stage of the case to excite the curative reaction. But his aim of emphasizing on applying lower potencies is not to render us inclined to their indiscriminate use, because there are, on the other hand, certain cases that can be cured only by highly potentiated preparations such as 10M, 50M, CM or higher.

From all the above quotes and discussion we deduce the following conclusive points:

1. We should use maximum range of potencies. The more extensive the armamentarium the more cases are cured. If we limit ourselves to some limited range of potencies, be they low, medium or high, we would be losing our powerful tools of practice and thus depriving our patients of valuable means of cure. Physicians who know how to use maximum range of potencies cure many times more patients than those who use a few potencies. Mostly in a stopped case the same remedy starts improving the patient again in a different potency. So never change the remedy until the patient is getting better under it. When an applied potency stops working try a higher potency before changing the remedy. That is, change the potency before changing the remedy. Also do not change potency until the patient is improving by the same.

2. Usually an applied potency works twice or maximum thrice and then we have to change it going to a higher potency.

3. Individualization is a must principle of homoeopathy; it is must not only for the selection of medicine but also the potency. Every patient has a different level of sensitivity and a different stage and seat of disease. Different degrees of potencies are likely more useful to different types of patients and their conditions. So, all degrees of potencies should be used according to the conditions and circumstances peculiar to them.

4. We should have all well-proved remedies in 6X, 12X, 6, 12, 30, 200, 1M, 10M, 50M and CM potencies for our usual practice.

5. Occasionally we may need the lowest potencies such as 3X or even mother tincture. Susceptibility in patients of greatly advanced pathologies and terminal conditions is very low and highly diluted preparations of homoeopathic medicines, some times, do not excite

reaction in them. In such cases we may resort to the lowest potencies.

6. On the other hand some times we may need the highest potencies such as CM, MM, 2MM and so on. Whenever we start a case from 10M or 50M (regarding the conditions) and the patient needs to be kept under the same remedy for a long time, there we would need highest potencies one after other ascending wise.

7. Fifty Millesimal Scale is Hahnemann's finally designed and recommended method of preparation and application of homoeopathic remedies. Potencies made on this scale also should be tried, for this scale has been reported of producing excellent results. Main advantage of this scale is minimum or no chances of homoeopathic aggravation in acute as well as chronic cases. These potencies can be applied on small children and sensitive women without danger of aggravation. Their action starts gently and goes on towards cure smoothly.

8. 1M, 10M and 50M can be initially applied in chronic cases, when (a) the remedy picture is very clear (b) the patient is not oversensitive and (c) there is no severe pathology. When the remedy picture is not clear our selection may be wrong; and when a wrong medicine is applied in a high potency, it may start unfavorable changes for a long time and thus the case may be spoiled. Higher potencies usually cause severe aggravation in oversensitive patients. They do not bear the aggravation and leave the treatment. So avoid high potencies in oversensitive patients (sensitive women and children). High potencies may also cause dangerous aggravation in severe pathological conditions such as suppuration in the liver or lungs. Aggravation of high potencies in such cases may be threatening even for the life of patient.

The Appropriate Potency

9. 200, 1M and 10M are suitable for acute cases with the same conditions that is, when (a) the remedy picture is very clear (b) the patient is not oversensitive and (c) there is no severe pathology.
10. When the remedy picture is not sufficiently clear 30 or 200 are best to start with both in acute and chronic cases.
11. In a case made confused by the use of many homoeopathic remedies we would have to give the best-selected remedy in a high potency (say 10M or 50M) and then allow it a considerable time to bring forth its results. We know that homoeopathic medicines produce very deep changes in the organism. When a case is confused by homoeopathic medicines, a high potency (of a very carefully selected remedy) can reach the disturbance and bring back the order. But it would require a long time, approximately 2-3 months to bring forth its clear result.
12. Oversensitive patients, especially sensitive women and children, should initially be given 30 or 200 in order to avoid undesirable and unbearable aggravation. When they get better under lower or medium potencies they will be able to receive (safely) high potencies.
13. Allopathically suppressed cases also should be started with 30 or 200. High potencies usually cause severe and prolonged aggravations in such cases.
14. Old and constitutionally weak patients should not be given high potencies at the start. Such patients have a poor reaction. When they receive too high a potency, it goes very deep into the organism which is incapable of producing curative reaction against it. In this way very high potency may happen to work, in such patients, like disease producing agent. That is, it starts its proving and producing its own symptoms in them. High potency of a similar remedy in old and constitutionally weak patients increases the suffering and hastens the end.

15. In case of advanced pathology deep remedies like Phosphorus and Sulphur, also nosodes (especially Medorrhinum), should not be given in high potencies. 30 or 200 are sufficient to start with. Deep and powerful remedies may cause severe, prolonged and even irreversible aggravation in such cases.

16. On the other hand some medicines are dangerous to use in very low potencies and repeated doses in cases of advanced pathologies. For example, 3X or 6X of Belladonna in case of meningitis and 6X or 12X of Phosphorus in case of severe pneumonia can be fatal. These medicines in such cases repeated in too low a potency can tear off the affected organ and take the patient's life. So 30 or 200 of these medicines would be suitable in such cases.

17. In cases of less advanced pathologies nosodes and other intercurrent remedies, if needed, should be given in comparatively high potencies (200, 1M, or 10M). Mostly we need nosodes in chronic miasmatic cases. So a deeper potency of a nosode often brings better result. But if there is sever pathology and we are going to apply a nosode, we would not go too high in order to avoid dangerous aggravation. There 30 or 200 would be sufficient.

18. In certain terminal conditions where medium and high potencies produce no reaction we may need to resort to the lowest preparations such as 3X, 1X or even material doses.

    In terminal conditions senses and internal function become slow; susceptibility and reaction decreases in proportion to the advancement of pathology. So lesser the susceptibility lower the potency.

19. High potencies correspond better to active people, intellectuals who are quick to act and react. Intellectuals like professors, teachers, and social workers etc. are mentally active; and those who take exercise and their

health is comparatively good, are physically active. So these people respond well to high potencies.

20. Low potencies are appropriate to dull people, sluggish mentally and physically, slow to act and react.

   Lower potencies and larger and frequent doses correspond better to torpid and phlegmatic individuals, dull of comprehension and slow to act; to coarse fibered, sluggish individuals of gross habits. People who have to work in the sun, work in factories and odors of chemicals and perfume sellers often need lower potencies and frequent doses.

21. We may use higher potencies when we have clear and characteristic symptoms. But if there are only common, pathological and local symptoms we shall apply lower potency. It is commonly said in homoeopathic circles that in cases with mental symptoms we should use high potencies. This is also because a remedy is confirmed when its mental symptoms are clear. But if there are only such mental symptoms which do not clearly fit into a particular remedy, high potency should not be used. Moreover if there are clear mental symptoms but other circumstances are not favorable for high potencies, we should avoid them.

22. The more active (physically and mentally) the patient the higher the potency and the weaker the patient the lower the potency. Strong and active patients can bear homoeopathic aggravations. Moreover reaction of their vital force against the similar remedy is strong. So we may use high potencies in strong individuals (but not dull).

23. Patient's physical and constitutional make-up, stage and condition of disease or other internal and external factors, whatever be the reasons, when reaction is low potency should be low and when reaction is strong and high, potency should be high.

24. When an applied potency does not work, after reconsidering the case we may choose another potency by going up or low. However when a potency has relieved a patient for a while but further it is not working and remedy is still the same, we shall proceed to higher potencies according to Kent's series of degrees e.g. 12X after 6X, or 12 after 6. Similarly 200 after 30 then 1M then 10M and so on.

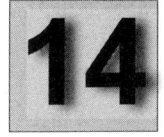

DOSE
Administration of Medicine

After reading typescript of this book a homoeopath friend, Dr. Kathy Thomas from New Zealand, suggested me to include into it a chapter on "Dose". Her suggestion seemed to be fit because a large percentage of failures occur only due to improper "Dose". When I studied the topic deeply it revealed to me that most homoeopaths, especially around me, were not aware of the proper way of dispensing homoeopathic medicines and this was one of major reasons of their failures in chronic cases.

Those so-called homoeopaths who apply non-sense combinations are not concerned here because they are not bound to any principle. They can mix any number of medicines in a vial and give repeatedly many drops of 1M and CM of deep remedies, like Sulphur and Medorrhinum, to their patients to shorten their journey to death. We are addressing here those honest beginners who select single remedy on the totality of symptoms and sincerely wish to cure the suffering human fellows.

Most single remedists in our country follow the "single dose wait and watch" method of Kent which he learned from the initial editions of the Organon. But this method causes two major difficulties in practice. Firstly it takes too long time to cure chronic diseases. Kent says in "Lesser Writings",

"When we recognize the fact of the long years of existence of chronic diseases, also that they are often inherited for several generations, if a cure is made in the course of two or three years it is indeed a speedy cure. It takes from two to five years to cure chronic diseases."

(J.T. Kent, Lesser Writings. P. 685)

On the other hand, Hahnemann says,

"But in more chronic diseases, on the other hand, a single dose of an appropriately selected homoeopathic remedy will at times complete even with slowly progressive improvement and give the help which such a remedy in such a case can accomplish naturally within 40, 50, 60 or 100 days. This is, however, but rarely the case; and besides, it must be a matter of great importance to the physician as well as to the patient that were it possible, this period should be diminished to one-half, one-quarter and even still less, so that a much more rapid cure might be obtained".

(Hahnemann, Organon, Aphorism 246, PP.270-71)

That is, a medicine in a chronic case should accomplish its beneficial action between 40 to 100 days. This period, too, can be rendered one-half, one-quarter or even lesser. It means according to Hahnemann if a chronic case requires 2-3 or 4-5 remedies, after one another, it will not take more than some months to complete the cure. Kent, two to five years; Hahnemann, a few months. It is a huge difference. The basic reason for this difference is that Kent used to work on Hahnemann's initial "single dose wait and watch" method. But Hahnemann was not satisfied with this method. He continued his experiments to improve homoeopathic posology more and more. Kent could not utilize Hahnemann's improved methods because he passed away in 1916 whereas Hahnemann's 6th Organon could be published in 1921 in which he introduced LM potencies and made marvelous changes in the posology. Kent could not utilize the results of most ripe experiments of Hahnemann and his most effective methods of adjusting the dose. Now we, single remedists, ought to think should we stick to the old method in which there are many difficulties or adopt those advanced methods where there are little chances of aggravations and chronic cases are cured comparatively in very short time. According to our observation reason for small percentage of cure in chronic cases in the hands of single remedists is the "single dose wait and watch" method. Since only one dose is given in this method, most homoeopaths use higher potencies, in order to speed up the case. The high potencies tend to cause severe aggravations particularly in hypersensitive and weak patients with deep pathologies. Hahnemann tried high potencies that caused problem of aggravations as we see, today, in the hands of high potency users. Some times even after the aggravation the required curative process does not start. Hahnemann says about high potencies,

"Thus increasing the strength of the single doses of the homoeopathic medicine with the view of effefcing the degree of pathogenetic excitation of the vital force necessary to produce satisfactory salutary reaction, fails altogether, as experience teaches, to accomplish the desired object. This vital force is there by too violently and too suddenly assailed and excited to allow it time to exercise a gradual equable, salutary reaction, to adapt itself to the modifications effected in it; hence it strikes to repel, as if it were an enemy".

(Hahnemann, Organon, Dudgeon P. 124)

So due to the aggravation by a high potency either patients leave the treatment at start, or later if the recovery is slow. Obviously when the patient has suffered much increase of symptoms and there is no significant improvement the result would be despair. I do not mean that all cases cause problems with high potencies. Certainly there are number of cases that are easily cured by high potencies .So I do not mean to oppose high potencies, rather to find the solution for such cases as are not tackled this way. Homoeopaths who prescribe on the totality of the symptoms and use high potencies usually fail because their potency, dose and repetition do not suit the case in hand.

When in order to avoid the aggravation we reduce the size of dose to one small globule or lesser it does not generate the required curative action .One small dry globule touches only a few nerves and does not influence the vital force effectively. Hahnemann says,

"Yet that in many, indeed in most cases, not only of very chronic diseases that have already made great progress and have frequently been aggravated by previous employment of inappropriate medicines, but also of serious acute diseases, one such smallest dose of medicine in our highly potentized dynamization is evidently insufficient to effect all the curative action that might be expected from that medicine... the best chosen medicine in such a small dose, given but once might certainly be of some service ,but would not be nearly sufficient".

(Hahnemann, Organon, Dudgeon, P. 123)

When such smallest dose does not serve the required curative action and high potencies create aggravation problem, the next option comes to increase the size of dose. Hahnemann made experiments on this, too, and the results were not satisfying. When we give 6-7 or 8 globules instead of one, or a few drops of the potency it becomes damaging instead of benefiting to the patient, and such damage is usually irreparable according to the master,

"And, for instance, in place of giving a single very minute globule moistened with the medicine in the highest dynamization, to administer six, seven or eight of them at once, and even a half or a whole drop. But the result was almost always less favorable than it should have been; it was often actually unfavorable, often even very bad---an injury that, in a patient so treated, it is difficult to repair".

(Hahnemann, Organon, Dudgeon, P. 124)

Thus increasing size of the dose even in highly potentized form could not serve better results. I have recently heard of a homoeopath who handovers the whole vial of 1M and even

CM potency to the patient and advises to take 5-10 drops continuously. Some homoeopaths drop the potency directly on patient's tongue. All this is due to lack of knowledge and training. They hope to achieve better effects by increasing size of the dose. But in fact the more similar the medicine the lesser the dose would be needed. And well-selected similar medicine in large doses causes more damage than benefit. Homoeopathic medicine in large doses, even potentized, takes place of the disease symptoms. That is, while curing the disease symptoms the medicine produces its own symptoms which are similar to the original ones. Now the patient is feeling nearly the same symptoms but they are produced by medicine not by the disease. At the same time such symptoms are so powerful as might never be eradicated. Luckily medicines given by such poor prescribers are not similar enough. If a truly similar medicine were given in such large quantities, only a few doses of it would be enough to render the patient incurable forever. When the medicine is given single, according to the law, there may be some possibility of antidoting it or expiring itself by the time. But I have seen people giving a number of mixed potentized medicines in large quantities as 5,10,15, or 20 drops many times a day; vial after vial is used up this way. Cases spoiled by large number of mixed medicines, affecting the same pathology, in such large quantities can never be cured.

Some homoeopaths think that action of medicine depends on degree of potency and quantity does not matter. They believe that action of one globule or many of them or even many drops of a potency would be the same. This is Kent's understanding who interpreted homoeopathic potencies as "simple substance" in which quantity does not concern. But the founder viewed potencies as "quantum energies" and the quantity can be divided and minimized as far as needed. We ought to make experiments. If 8-10 globules of a 1M or 10M potency cause sever aggravation, there would be minimum or no aggravation if we take one globule of the same preparation, dissolve it into a cup of water and give one or half spoonful to the patient as a dose. Hahnemann's observations were deeper. No one equals the master. He says even giving more succussions to the same potency enhance its energy. The more succussions we give the more powerful is the dilution,

"In order to maintain a fixed and measured standard for developing the power of liquid medicines, multiplied experience and careful observation have led me to adopt two succussions for each phial, in preference to the greater number formerly employed (by which medicine were too highly potentized). There are, however, homoeopathists who carry about with them on their visits to patients the homoeopathic medicines in fluid state, and who yet assert that they do not become more highly potentized in the course of time, but they there by show their want of ability to observe correctly. I dissolved a grain of soda in half ounce of water mixed with alcohol in a phial, which was thereby filled two – thirds full, and shook this solution continuously for half an hour, and this fluid was in potency and energy equal to the thirtieth development of power":

(Hahnemann, Organon, Dudgeon PP. 135-36)

If the dose is greatly minimized it does not produce the required action; if the potency is greatly raised it causes severe aggravations; and if the size of dose is increased it causes adverse effects. Then what would be the way to attain "rapid, gentle and permanent" cure. Perhaps repetition; repeating the medicine in comparatively lower potency and smaller doses. Hahnemann made experiments on this option, also, and the results again were not satisfying. If the first dose effected some favorable changes the later doses (of the same potency in the same size of dose) did not further improve the case, rather the later doses, which were equal in degree and size to the former, reversed the improvement made by the first dose. Hahnemann says when several same doses are repeated they accumulate in the system and then their effects are like that of a very large dose. And it is evident that large doses of a similar medicine are injurious.

"But it happens, moreover, that a number of smallest doses given for the same object in quick succession accumulate in the organism into a kind of excessively large dose, with (a few rare cases excepted) similar bad results".

(Hahnemann, Organon, Dudgeon, P. 124)

It means repeating the same dose (same in degree and size) can cure a small percentage of cases. Although homoeopaths who repeat 30 or 6X in a routine way cure some cases but their percentage is very small. And we, being homeopaths, ought to serve people with the maximum cures. So what should we do for such cases as do not respond to repetition in a better way. If the dose is very small (as one or two small dry globules given only once) it does not start curative action. If potency is too high, in order to obtain curative action from such a small dose, it causes aggravations. If the potency is not very high but the size of dose is too large, it produces its bad effects in form of proving like symptoms. If the size of dose is very small and it is repeated, it accumulates in the organism and the effects are like that of a large dose. Although some cases are cured by each of these techniques yet collective percentage remains still very small. These were problems for which Hahnemann continued his experiments on homoeopathic posology and after all he discovered such methods as served him to attain "rapid, gentle and permanent" cure by homoeopathic medicines.

First change in this respect was the founder's conversion, in his 5th Organon, from "single dose wait and watch" method to repeated doses. I think necessary to mention here that in spite of this conversion to repeated doses Hahnemann maintained the principle of not repeating medicine in cases strikingly and speedily improving by single dose.

"Every perceptibly progressive and strikingly increasing amelioration in a transient (acute) or persistent (chronic) disease, is a condition as long as it lasts, completely precludes every repetition of the administration of any medicine whatsoever, because all the good the medicine taken continues to effect is now hastening towards its completion".

(Hahnemann, Organon, Dudgeon aphorism 245, P. 122)

When a case starts improving speedily and strikingly, either acute or chronic, it would need no repetition. It means like selection of medicine and potency administration of medicine would also be individualized for every patient. The most important point in "repeated doses method " is that Hahnemann did not allow blind continuous repetition. He conditioned it with "suitable intervals" and the intervals would be adjusted on the basis of duration of action of the fist dose that may be different in every case according to patient's temperament, origin of the medicine, chosen potency as well as stage and condition of the disease. For instance, if a dose of Sulphur 30 continues improving a case for 5 days and from 6th day symptoms are relapsing, the dose should be repeated at every 4th day until the patient gets well. Similarly when a dose of Sulphur 30 works for 10 days the dose would be repeated at every 9th day. Hahnemann says,

"The dose of the same medicine may be repeated several times according to circumstances, but only so long as until either recovery ensues, or the same remedy ceases to do good and the rest of the disease, presenting a different group of symptoms, demand a different homoeopathic remedy".

(Hahnemann, Organon Dudgeon, Aphorism 248, P.127)

In this respect Hahnemann has given detailed instructions in aphorism 246 and its footnote of the 5th Organon .He suggested there to observe three factors in order to achieve a speedy cure. (1) The remedy should be the best similar (2) It should be highly potentized. (3) It should be repeated at "suitable intervals". Whereas in the 6th edition he added, in the light of his many years experiments, two more conditions (1) the dose should be dissolved in water (2) and every dose must be more potentized (raised in degree) than the previous one,

"And this may be very happily affected, as recent and oft-repeated observations have taught me under the following conditions firstly, if the medicine selected with utmost care was perfectly homoeopathic, secondly if it is highly potentized, dissolved in water and given in proper small dose that experience has taught as the most suitable and in definite interval for the quickest accomplishment of the cure but with precaution, that the degree of every dose deviate somewhat from the preceding and following in order that the vital principle which is to be altered to a similar medicinal disease be not aroused to unwanted reactions and revolt as is always the case with un modified and especially rapidly repeated doses".

(Hahnemann, Organon 6th Aphorism 246, P. 271)

If the dose is too small (one or two smallest globules) it makes very little influence on the body. The master solved this problem by dissolving the same dose into water. Thus the dose touches more internal parts of the body, than one small globule, and becomes more effective and capable of bringing required changes. Secondly if repetition is necessary every next dose must be more potentized than the former one. Next full aphorism (247) explains this point that only first dose of the medicine acts on similar symptoms and all the following doses start (as dry pellets or liquid not further succussed) producing medicinal symptoms. To say more clearly the first dose acts on the similar symptoms whereas the following doses start developing such symptoms of the applied medicine as the patient not had before. But when the medicine is given in liquid form and every later dose is further succussed, 8 to 10 times, it becomes little higher in degree of potentization and every following dose acts on the similar symptoms curatively. In this way the indicated remedy can be repeated as long as needed or till the symptoms picture changes and a new remedy is indicated.

Single dose of a high potency makes a sudden turmoil in the organism and then exhausts without producing long lasting effects (a few cases exempted). This action resembles that of acute diseases and we see that this mode of administration of medicine works better in acute and sub-chronic diseases particularly when the disease is mostly on functional level. On the other hand mild, modified and repeated doses start bringing changes in a mild way and keep on bringing changes in the organism. This mode of action is similar to the nature and progression of chronic diseases. Experience shows that these Hahnemann's lastly introduced wonderful techniques of administration of medicine are the best and final solution to cure chronic diseases. Each mild and modified dose makes a little more change and the case continuously, smoothly and speedily runs towards cure.

Another must notable point in this aphorism is that the master said "definite intervals" (in the 6th Organon) instead of "suitable intervals" (5th Organon). It means when the case does not significantly start improving by single dose or giving the medicine at longer intervals we would continuously have to keep the patient under the influence of medicine; that is, to repeat the medicine at regular/definite intervals as long as some clear change is noticed. Hahnemann suggests repeating medicine, in this way, in chronic cases daily or every other day, in acute cases after two or six hours and in extreme emergency every hour or as shorter intervals as required. It is to be remembered that in spite of advocating repetition Hahnemann maintained the principle of single dose when the case starts strikingly and progressively improving by it. When we have to continuously repeat the medicine every following dose should be a little more potentized than the preceding one. In order to fully understand Hahnemann's advanced method of water doses and repetition of step by step potentized medicine we should carefully read through his aphorisms 246-48 and their footnotes of the 6th Organon.

Briefly, for this purpose, we would take 8, 15, 20, 30, or 40 tablespoonfuls of distilled water with a little quantity of alcohol and dissolve into it one (some times two or more) small medicated globule. Then succuss this medicinal solution 8-10 times and give one spoonful to the patient as a dose. Before ingesting every dose the solution must be again succussed 8,10 or 12 times. If one spoonful does not work we can increase the dose to two or more spoonful as required. In this way we can repeat every day, even long acting medicines, for weeks and months; but only when and as necessary.

For hypersensitive patients the medicinal solution can be made more and more mild according to the level of their sensitivity. For this purpose we would take one teaspoonful of the medicinal solution (made of one or two globules dissolved in 7-8 tablespoons of water and succussed 8,10 or 12 times) and again mix it into further 7-8 spoonful of water. Then stir it sufficiently and give, from this 2nd solution, one spoonful as a dose. This procedure can be repeated to 3rd, 4th or 5th solution according to suitability of case in hand. Children can be given one-half, infants one-quarter spoon of the first, or second or the required solution. Every time such a dose is to be taken it should be prepared a new from the first medicinal solution after giving it 8, 10, or 12 powerful, succussions. The globule before dissolving should be grinded with a few grains of sugar of milk. In chronic cases one potency (LM1, LM2, 6C, 12C or 30C) can be continued for one or two weeks and then next higher potency should be started if necessary. In this way the patient can be kept under the influence of an indicated remedy as long as it continues improving. If in this course of repetition new symptoms develop, it means the case has moved to a new direction and then another, more similar, remedy should be sought and repeated according to the prescribed method. It is to be remembered that every next dose must be a little more potentized than the former.

High potencies and large doses (dry globules) often produce aggravation at the start of administering a medicine whereas mild and very minute doses (diluted water doses) mostly initiate improvement without causing any aggravation. If a first water dose too causes aggravation we shall give a second more diluted dose from the second glass; if this too aggravates then a third dose from the next glass will be given.

This prcedure is particularly required in deep pathological cases where repetition and even application of a single dose of an indicated medicine brings aggravation. Hahnemann made experiments on this formulation for many years and after being satisfied with it he adopted the procedure of applying mild water doses which were repeated when and as necessary.

In some cases homoeopathic aggravation occurs after repeating the medicine for some period. It means that similar medicinal symptoms have taken place of the disease symptoms. In this condition the medicine should be stopped or repeated at longer intervals (as required for the case). When the symptoms do not relapse, after stopping the medicine, it means the case needs no more medication. Hahnemann, in the 6th Organon, ascribed water-doses to his lastly introduced LM potencies. However in last years practice he applied both centesimal and fifty-millesimal scales in water doses.

For extraordinary or ultra-hypersensitive patients we can apply medicine through olfaction. Dr. Pierre Schmidt describes in his booklet "The Art of Case Taking" a case of a boy who had clear-cut symptoms of Lycopodium but an oral dose of the 200th potency caused a severe aggravation. They waited for several days but the aggravation did not subside, then they gave an olfaction dose of 10,000 potency that promptly cured the boy. Hahnemann was great; he was true to tell that the best homoeopathic dose is the least possible. For preparing the olfaction dose we would dissolve one globule, of the indicated remedy and potency, into one or two drops of water, then fill the vial two third with pure alcohol and give it 8 to 12 succussions. The patient should smell this medicated solution through one or both nostrils, as required, as a dose. If more doses are needed, every dose should be smelt after giving the vial 8 to 10 more succussions.

Now we present some cases from our record book to highlight the necessity and utility of Hahnemann's last gift to the homoeopathic profession----the water doses.

Cases 1

A delicate girl of 15 years was brought to us for treatment of epilepsy. She was suffering from epileptic convulsions from 2 months. An allopathic physician had put her on Epival, an anti-convulsive drug. The drug controlled her convulsions but she was constantly feeling laziness and weakness. She was seized with the convulsions after allopathic treatment of fever and coryza. Her fits became worse during menses. She felt tremendous fear of death before a fit and cried due to this fear. There was great anxiety before the fit. There were troublesome vertigos before and during the fit. Beside convulsions we obtained the following symptoms. Trembling of extremities which caused difficulty in writing and handling things. Irritability and anger, trembling of extremities with anger, trembling of extremities < when talking to her teacher and in the examination hall. Desire for salt things and cold drinks. Heaviness of shoulders after waking in the morning. Weeping inclination with consolation aggravation.

She suffered from trembling of extremities after a dreadful incident in their home. She had headache which was agg. during reading. She had fear of dark and fear of being alone.

After repertorizing and studying the case Arg-n was selected. Since she was taking an anti-convulsive drug it was decided to repeat the medicine at definite intervals instead of single dose wait and watch method. Arg-n 6C one dose at night before going to sleep was started on 13-02-11. Her medicine was prepared by dissolving one dry globule (10 Number) of Arg-n 6C into fifteen tablespoons of distilled water and thirty drops of alcohol.

First follow up after fifteen days dated 28-02-11

Fits markedly decreased, only one fit occurred in fifteen days, trembling of extremities aggravated. Her coryza, which had been stopped by allopathic medicines, re-established. A beautiful action of the remedy! If she were not taking allopathic drugs her remedy should have been stopped at that point.

Prescription: Arg-n 6C from 2nd glass was continued and the anti-convulsive drug was reduced to half.

Follow up dated 12-03-11

No fit in fifteen days, vertigo almost ended, coryza and heaviness of head did not decrease.

Prescription: Arg-n 6C from 3rd glass, anti-convulsive drug stopped.

Follow up dated 26-03-11

Vertigo relapsed, one fit in fifteen days.

Prescription: Arg-n 1M single dose with placebo for fifteen days.

Follow up dated 11-04-11

Only one fit in fifteen days but vertigos increased. Vertigos were amel. by lying and agg. in the dark. On 20-04-11 she had a severe fit after suddenly hearing news of her friend's death.

Prescription: Arg-n LM1 one dose daily. She was also advised to restart Epival to immediately control the fits.

Follow up dated 09-05-11

No fit in fifteen days, over all condition also better.

Prescription: Arg-n LM1 one dose daily from second glass. When the remedy controlled the condition she was also advised to reduce the anti-convulsive drug to half.

Follow up dated 22-05-11

Only one fit in fifteen days, which occurred during menses. However it was notably milder than previous ones. Vertigos increased from 2-3 days and her head felt heavy.

Prescription: Placebo. Advised to stop anti-convulsive drug. Also advised to restart Arg-n LM1 from second glass in condition of relapsing symptoms.

Follow up dated 04-06-11

No fit, vertigos also decreased.
Prescription: Placebo.

Follow up dated 19-06-11

No fit, vertigos steadily decreasing, health improving.
Prescription: Placebo.

Follow up dated 03-07-11

Vertigos again increased. On questioning it was informed that vertigos increased on returning from her tour with family to mountain areas. But it did not decrease while she was at home from 5-6 days.
Prescription: Arg-n LM1, one dose daily from third glass.

Follow up dated 31-07-11

Vertigos somewhat decreased, no fit. That month she developed pustular eruptions on her face. Gradually the eruptions were increasing and the vertigos decreasing.
Prescription: Placebo.

Follow up dated 28-08-11.

No fit, vertigos ended, eruptions also decreased. Over all health greatly improved.

Interpretation

The patient was taking a powerful anti-convulsive allopathic drug and it was not possible for homoeopathic medicine to work on her with "single dose wait and watch" method.

Arg-n 6C given in water doses at definite intervals brought very good changes. When the allopathic drug was completely stopped a single dose of the well-selected remedy in 1M potency could not effect lasting improvement. However the same remedy given in LM potency and repeated at definite intervals speedily cured the case.

Case 2

A lady of 33 years came to us for treatment of certain complaints. She had the following symptoms and complaints.

Pain in throat < talking, hoarseness, mucus in throat, cough and lumps of mucus expelled by coughing, constriction of throat, painful dry cough, pain in muscles, hair falling out speedily, backache lumber and sacral region < stooping and lying, profuse perspiration worse on face, neck and back. Generally she was sensitive to both heat and cold, warm drinks amel. her complaints particularly of throat.

She had born two children by c-section. She had a history of typhoid in her childhood. A few years ago she consulted allopathic physicians for the above mentioned complaints. They diagnosed hypothyroidism for which she had been taking Thyroxin for 2 years. That time she had a strong desire for sweets which decreased afterwards.

After repertorizing and studying the case Lycopodium was selected and given in 6C potency. The medicine was prepared by dissolving one dry globule (10 number) into 15 spoons of distilled water. The patient was advised to take one spoonful of the medicinal solution at bedtime and give 8-10 succussions to the bottle before ingesting each dose.

Telephone report dated 15-04-11

All the symptoms aggravated, fever with drawing of tongue, the whole body seemed powerless, weakness was so extreme as she could not wink her eyes, cough was so severe as she could not talk due to it. She was advised to stop the medicine.

Two days after the aggravation was same and troubling the patient very much. So she was advised to take the medicine from second glass. Two days after still she was feeling bad yet the aggravation was decreasing. Then she was advised to take half a spoonful from fourth glass. On 25-04-11 all symptoms markedly decreased and she was feeling well. On 05-05-11 she had some hoarseness and pain in throat. On questioning it was revealed that she took very cold water. She was given placebo and advised to take some warm drinks and avoid cold ones. On 22-05-11 she reported that all her symptoms had ended. She is well till the time of writing.

Interpretation

One tablespoonful dose from first solution of 6C potency caused much aggaravation. If the patient were given several globules of a high potency she would have to suffer severe aggravation for a long time. If the remedy were repeated in long intervals the case would have taken too long time to be cured. But when the remedy was applied in mild water doses at regular intervals, according to the final instructions of Hahnemann, the chronic case was cured in a period less than two months. When the aggravation occurred and the medicine was stopped, the aggravation did not subside until the medicine was repeated in milder and more diluted doses. When the dose was significantly reduced to half a spoon from the fourth glass both the aggravation and the original symptoms ended in a few days.

Case 3

A 30 years lady was ill from several years. Her sufferings had been gradually increasing and she was in the worst condition from two months. Allopathic doctors made many tests but could neither detect nor diagnose any disease. After all a physician suggested her to resort to some spiritual treatment. From 2-3 months she was suffering from a painful constriction in her head which was troubling her very much. She also had the following symptoms. Noises in ears, sensitiveness to noises, sinking of heart with palpitation. She was suffering form blurred vision from 18 months which occurred from time to time. With this blurred vision and sinking of heart her face used to become blackish. Five years ago she had a tumor on a side of uterus which had been removed by operation. Her feet remained cold. In general symptoms she was sensitive to cold, angry and irritable. During the complaints she wished to be let alone. It was an important point in this case that before her marriage she had tedious fever for many years. The fever had left her from some years but afterwards the above-mentioned complaints had made her life miserable.

After repertorizing the case China 30 was prescribed. A medicinal solution was prepared by dissolving one dry globule of China 30 into 8 spoons of distilled water and 30 drops of alcohol. The patient was advised to take a dose of one spoonful daily giving 8-10 succussions to the medicinal solution before ingesting each dose.

She started the medicine on 12-07-11 and till 19-07-11 all symptoms severely aggravated. Her appetite also decreased. Then she was advised to take one spoonful daily from second glass. After taking first dose from the second glass the aggravation subsided. But the next day symptoms relapsed. One spoonful direct from the medicinal solution caused severe aggravation whereas a spoonful dose from the second glass could not overcome the symptoms. Logically she was advised to take a spoonful daily from first glass. (One spoonful of the medicinal solution mixed into 4 ounces of drinking water and after stirring it well one spoonful of it as a dose) It adjusted to the patient well and stared speedy improvement. The day of 25-07-11 was a pleasant time in her life after many years. All the day she felt very well and free of all symptoms. On 26-07-11 she again felt slight return of symptoms. Then the medicine was stopped. On 27-07-11 aphthae reappeared in her mouth that she had many years ago. She was given placebo, no medicine for the aphthae. She did not come afterwards. Certainly she did not need to come because she was cured.

Interpretation

One spoonful of the medicinal solution caused severe aggravation whereas a spoonful of the second glass could not overcome the symptoms. However a spoonful of the first glass made a speedy cure.

In this way by decreasing or increasing quantity of the dose and repeating it at definite intervals we can achieve speedy cures. If a given dose aggravates we should decrease it by diluting it more and more until it adjusts the sensitivity of our patient. On the other hand when a given dose does not produce desired changes we can speed up the case by increasing its quantity and repetition. Once I applied Calc-c LM1 on a patient. Medicinal solution for the patient was prepared by dissolving one globule of Calc-c LM1 into 15 tablespoons of distilled water of which the patient was to take one spoonful at bedtime. No marked improvement happened in a week. So the patient was advised to take a dose of two spoonfuls daily. From the very second day of starting 2 spoonfuls as a dose improvement started. In another case of epilepsy Belladonna 30 was given. Medicinal solution was prepared by dissolving one dry globule of the medicine into 30 spoons of distilled water. The patient was advised to take a dose of one spoonful daily. The epileptic fits did not decrease in one month however slight improvement was felt in other symptoms. Then the patient was advised to take one spoonful twice a day. After 15 days the patient was feeling better and the fits also became less frequent. In this way we can achieve rapid, gentle and permanent cures by decreasing or increasing quantity and repetition of the dose. Salute to Hahnemann for his painstaking discoveries and devoting his all life to the mankind. The artistic and highly valuable method of "water doses" is the ripe fruit of old age of our great master.

STUDY OF REPERTORY

Repertory is a great source for enhancing our knowledge of Materia Medica. By constant study and use of repertory we come to know such symptoms of remedies that are not described in small or filtered books of Materia Medica. By and by our knowledge of Materia Medica is increased and we come to know the use of different remedies in different diseased conditions according to their varied symptoms. Moreover while consulting a rubric for some case we come across such remedies that are not in our knowledge before. Then we study those remedies also and retain them in mind for day to day practice. Dr. Julia M. Green, M. D. says in an essay "Methods of studying Materia Medica". (Available on www.homeoint.org

"Then there are rich gems of materia medica knowledge to be found in perusing the repertory. The habit of thumbing through parts of Kent's Repertory, for instance, during scarce idle moments is an excellent habit. One acquires new slants on old remedy friends from finding these in a list where their appearance is real news, or finding a grading for a symptom which one did not know before. Or, hunting for a peculiar symptom, one finds it in a repertory list belonging to a drug never before associated with such a symptom. Or repertorial analysis of a case brings for study a small group of remedies with new lights on them often unsuspected even after many long years in homoeopathic practice."

Dr. Jugal Kishore says,

"The materia medica and repertory go hand in hand and nobody can master either of the subjects without referring to other. It has been found that great repertorians were also the masters of materia medica. Of course no repertory can be made or improved without constant study of our materia medicas. It is a hard a laborious study but the rewards are none the less as sweets".

(Jugal Kishore, Introduction, Kent's Lectures on Materia Medica, P. 9)

16

LITERATURE ON HOMOEOPATHIC MATERIA MEDICA

Books acquire importance according to the stage of our learning. One should start studying Homoeopathic Materia Medica from such books, which provide basic, essential and perfect knowledge in an easy and concise way. When the basic knowledge has been obtained and a familiarity with the subject has been generated, one can turn towards the main and important literature. As for the books of reference, we have to cultivate a sort of friendship, a familiarity of high degree, if we are to get from them the knowledge and information, we need for a full practice.

Keeping these points in mind we shall recommend the important books dividing them into three classes.

1. Elementary Stage.
2. Middle Stage.
3. Advanced stage.

Of course this is an arbitrary division, which is made only for the sake of convenience. Depending upon the depth of interest of the student and his speed of learning, he could firstly glance through the books in a library and then decide about those he would like to buy for his constant reference, irrespective of the categories or stages assigned here.

ELEMENTARY STAGE

(Books essential for beginners and new students)
With Organon of Medicine

1. Leaders in Homoeopathic Therapeutics.

   E.B. Nash

2. Homoeopathic Drug Picture

   M.L. Tyler.

3. Comparative Study on Kent's Materia Medica.

   A. Gaskin.

4. Key Notes of Leading Remedies.

   H.C. Allen

5. Genius of Homoeopathic Remedies

   Gunavante.

6. Pocket Manual of the Homoeopathic Materia Medica.

   W. Boericke.

7. Materia Medica of Homoepathic Medicines

   S.R. Phatak

MIDDLE STAGE

(Books essential for Secondary Students as well as clinical practice)
With Organon of Medicine

1. Lectures on Homoeopathic Materia Medica.

   J.T. Kent.

2. Clinical Materia Medica.

   E.A. Farrington.

3. Chronic Diseases (2Vols)

   Hahnemann.

4. Condensed Materia Medica.
   C. Hering.
5. Key Notes and Red Line Symptoms of The Homoeopathic Materia Medica
   A. V.Lippe
6. Systematic Materia Medica.
   K.N. Mathur.
7. Essence of Materia Medica.
   G. Vithoulkas.
8. Physiological Materia Medica.
   William Burt.
9. A Study on Materia Medica.
   N.M. Choudhuri
10. Key Notes of the Materia Medica, Commentary and Group Discussion.
    R. Murphy

ADVANCE STAGE

(Books for extensive study and reference work)

1. Hand Book of Materia Medica and Homoeopathic Therapeutics.
   T.F.Allen.
2. A Dictionary of Practical Materia Medica. (3Vols)
   J.H. Clarke.
3. The Guiding Symptoms of Our Materia Medica (10Vols)
   C. Hering.
4. Encyclopedia of Pure Materia Medica. (12Vols)
   T.F. Allen.
5. Materia Medica Pura.
   Hahnemann

STUDY PLAN

It is essential for the beginner to know that it is not necessary to read through all the Materia Medica books from beginning to end. These books comprise thousands of pages and it would definitely be very hard for a beginner to read, comprehend and retain such a huge bulk of text on a quite new subject.

Upon the initial reading of the prescribed Materia Medica books it is quite possible that the student will retain very little of the most important points. And the reading will not divulge which Homoeopathic remedies are used frequently and which ones are used rarely. So it is not clear upon a biginner how to proceed in the study. Such remedies as have been proved thoroughly and produced a lot of symptoms correspond to many common diseases and ailments. Hence they are frequently required in practice such as Arsenic, Bryonia, Calcarea, Carbo veg, Lycopodium, Merc Sol, Matrum mur, Pulsatilla and Sulphur etc. Acute remedies that help in common acute diseases are also used frequently such as Belladonna, Ipecac, and Gelsemium etc. On the other hand certain remedies have been proved partially and we know a few of their effects. Also there are medicines which have a limited sphere of action and their symptoms correspond to very rare conditions. We rarely need such medicines.

Therefore, firstly we should study and understand sufficiently the remedies which we will need frequently even at start of our practice. The more frequently used the remedy the more deep and thorough we need to understand it. So we have to read and re-read the frequently used remedies again and again. Every encounter we have with a remedy reveals its points and features new to us. This simply enhances our knowledge and understanding of it.

A deeply acting constitutional remedy cannot be completely understood and retained in the mind by reading it only once. We have to keep on studying the materia medica in a systematic way for a successful practice. All master prescribers, like Kent, had prepared their lists of selected remedies and used to read them repeatedly.

Keeping these factors in view we can adopt the following plan for the study of the homoeopathic materia medica. We should also keep in mind that this classification of remedies has been made only for convenience in the study. Selection in all acute and chronic diseases always will be according to the symptoms. We may need a chronic remedy for acute complaints according to the symptoms. Also an acute remedy may be required at start or during the treatment of a chronic disease.

1. First of all we should study such acute remedies that are frequently indicated in common acute ailments such as common colds, cough, disorders of stomach and bowels, fevers, nausea, vomiting and cholera etc. Although such small acute remedies are comparatively easy to understand yet it is necessary to be well acquainted with them.

LEVEL 1

Aconite, Allium cepa, Arnica, Belladonna, Bryonia, Chamomilla, Colocynth, Cuprum, Drosera, Euphrasia, Gelsemium, Ipecac, Nux-vomica, Rhus-tox, Veratrum alb.

2. Then we would study those well-proved and constitutional remedies which are mostly indicated in chronic diseases. Mostly people do not consult homoeopaths for acute emergencies. Rare or unusual

remedies are required only when the practice is considerably extended and the homoeopath has to face variety of chronic cases with advanced pathologies. So Calc, Ars, Lach, Lyco, Merc, Puls, Sil, Sulph and such common constitutional remedies are the most frequently used in homoeopathic practice. Remember to revise the first group while studying the second.

LEVEL 2

Aesculis hip, Aethusa, Aloe, Alumina, Antim crud, Antim-tart, Apis, Argentum nit, Arsenic Alb, Baryta carb, Berberis, Borex, Calcarea carb, Calcarea phos, Calcarea sulph, Calendula, Cantheris, Carbo veg, China, Cina, Caulophyllum, Dioscorea, Ferrum met, Ferrum phos, Graphites, Hepar sulph, Ignatia, Iodium, Kali carb, Kali phos, Kali sulph, Lachesis, Ledum, Lycopodium, Magnesia mur, Magnesia phos, Medorrhinum, Mercurius, Naja, Natrum carb, Natrum mur, Natrum sulph, Opium, Petroleum, Phosphoric acid, Phosphorus, Phytolacca, Podophyllum, Psorinum, Pulsatilla, Sabina, Sambucus nigra, Sanguinaria can, Sarsaparilla, Secale cor, Selenium, Sepia, Silicea, Spongia, Staphisagria, Stramonium, Sulphur, Syphyllinum, Thuja, Tuberculinum.

3. Now we would study the remedies that we need occasionally in our practice; very rare remedies still would not be concerned. Now again remedies of both the first and second groups would be included in the reading list in order to revise them and understand them more deeply and thoroughly.

When we would have learned and understood these 140 remedies we would have developed sufficient familiarity with the materia medica and would be able to study and understand what we would need or want. Now we would also be able to study one by one all books of the first (elementary) stage from start to end. In this way we would study and pay attention to all remedies appropriate to their status and value in the practice. The more frequently used remedies would be studied more repeatedly and understood more deeply and thoroughly.

It is also essential to write down all the important information and salient features of all remedies in a personal notebook.

LEVEL 3

Abrotanum, Agaricus, Ambra grasia, Ammonium carb, Ammonium mur, Anacardium, Apocynum, Arum triphyllum, Aurum met, Baptisia, Cactus, Calcarea fluor, Camphor, Carbo animalis, Carduus mar, Chelidonium, Cimicifuga, Cocculus indicus, Coffea, Colchicum, Conium, Crotton tig, Digitalis, Dulcamara, Eupatorium perf, Flouric acid, Glonoin, Hamamelis, Hecla lava, Hyoscyamus, Kali bi, Kali mur, Kalmia, Kreosotum, Lac def, Latrodectus mactans, Lillium tig, Magnesia carb, Merc cor, Mezerium, Moschus, Murex, Muriatic acid, Natrum phos, Nux moschata, Picric acid, Plantago major, Platinum, Pyrogenium, Rheum, Rhododendron, Sabadilla, Spigelia, Stannum, Sulphur iod, Symphytum, Tabacum, Tarentula hisp, Tarentula cub, Zincum met.

Remainder of the book consists of a sample study of remedies. Following the introduction to important mateira medicas and short biographies of their authors, I have included the original text of a complete sample remedy in order to introduce their method and style to the reader in an empirical way.

SAMPLE STUDY

Leaders in Homoeopathic Therapeutics

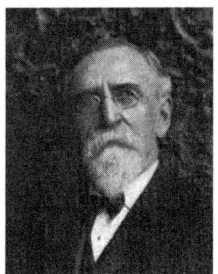

E.B. Nash

Eugene Beauharnias Nash was born on March 8th 1838 in Hillsdale Columbia County New York. He was one of America's leading 19th century homoeopaths. He graduated from Cleveland Homoeopathic Medical College in 1874. He served as Professor of Materia Medica in New York Homoeopathic Medical College for seven years. He was a member of the American Homoeopathic Society, of the New York State Homoeopathic Medical Society and an honorary member of the Pennsylvania State Homoeopathic Medical Society. In 1903 he became president of the International Hahnemannian Association (IHA). In 1905 he gave, by invitation, a course of lectures in the Homoeopathic Hospital of London. He authored the following books:

1. Directions for the Domestic Use of Homoeopathic Remedies.
2. Leaders in Homoeopathic Therapeutics.
3. Leaders in Typhoid Fever.
4. Leaders for the Use of Sulphur.
5. How to Take the Case and Find the Simillimum.
6. Leaders in Respiratory Organs.
7. The Testimony of Clinic.

Nash is considered one of the great teachers of the Homoeopathic Materia Medica. His "Leaders in Homoeopathic Therapeutics" is said to have converted many allopathic physicians to homoeopathy. There are a large number of Homoeopathic physicians in different parts of the world to day who owe their success in healing the sick to Nash's writings.

Nash's "Leaders in Homoeopathic Therapeutics" bears many qualities for which it should be prescribed as first Materia Medica reading for students of Homoeopathic Medicine. It is greatly useful for beginners. Its salient features are as under:

It is concise and easy. It seems that Nash, being an expert teacher of the Homoeopathic Materia Medica, intended to make it easily understandable and retainable for beginners and he hit the aim successfully. For the ease of beginners he especially regarded brevity. He says,

"Let us say here, that it is not our aim in this work to write exhaustively upon any remedy, but to point out a few of the chief virtues and characteristic symptoms, around which all the rest revolve."

(Nash, Leaders in Homoeopathic Therapeutics P. 21)

The second and very beautiful feature is its unique order in which it flows. Instead of typical alphabetical order Nash has grouped remedies respecting their relation to particular ailments that patients present to us. This provides us with a better understanding of remedies in connection to our daily practice. For example, he starts from Nux-v followed by Pulsatilla, Bryonia and Ant-c. --- remedies that generally correspond to digestive disorders. When a patient comes to us with a chief complaint of digestive problem, we can easily choose his remedy if he belongs to one of them. Sepia, Murex Purpurea, Lillium Tigrinum, Viburnum Opulus, Secale Cornutum, Caulophyllum, Actaea Racemosa, Sabina and Helonias have been grouped together as they chiefly affect female genital organs. Then we see Erigeron, Trillium and Millefolium three haemorrhagic remedies under one heading. Similarly Digitalis, Cactus, and Spigelia, that are chief heart remedies, come after each other. This is Nash's wonderful technique to teach Materia Medica in order to bring it into practice.

Another important quality is comparisons and contrasts of remedies which provide us with deep understanding of Materia Medica and enable us to pick out the most suitable remedy for the patient in hand. Let us read here some valuable comparisons,

"These are reliable symptoms, as given in Hering's cards, and are not very much like the symptoms of Nux vomica, which is not disturbed by fats, but on the contrary likes them and they agree. With Nux vomica warm food agrees best; with Pulsatilla, cold things."(Pulsatilla)

"How peculiar that Pulsatilla should have dry mouth and no thirst, while Mercurius should have characteristically moist mouth with intense thirst." (Pulsatilla)

(Nash, Leaders in Homoeopathic Therapeutics P. 25)

"The expectoration of Pulsatilla, which is thick, green and bland, tastes bitter, while that of Stannum is sweet and that of Kali hydroiodicum and Sepia salty."(Pulsatilla)

(Nash, Leaders in Homoeopathic Therapeutics P. 26)

"Belladonna may relieve the attack, but Aurum goes deeper and is more lasting in its effects. Aurum is one of our best remedies for bone pains. Never forget it. It ranks with Kali iodide, Asafoetida and the Mercurius in periosteal affections." (Aurum Metallicum)

(Nash, Leaders in Homoeopathic Therapeutics P. 293)

Along with describing important symptoms Nash gives us useful tips for daily practice extracted from his long experience of over 40 years.

Nash not only provides beginners with essential information of remedies but also warns against common mistakes in their use. This is why his followers start practice on right lines. Usually beginners, due to insufficient knowledge, follow partially understood concepts. Also there prevail many misconceptions in homoeopathy and many of our remedies are frequently misused. Nash strictly discourages to follow baseless and wrong concepts and thus helps beginners avoid mistakes and consequent failures at start of practice. Some examples of his knowledgeable advices are as under:

(i) "So no physician would be justified in prescribing Nux vomica on temperament alone, be the indication ever so clear. The whole case must come in."

(Nash, Leaders in Homoeopathic Therapeutics P. 15)

(ii) "It took me years to learn the value of this symptom, because I was a routinist and thought that Aconite, Belladonna, or both in alternation, must be given in all cases where high fever was present. So I have some sympathy for young physicians now, who from false teachings have been led into the same error. But let me say here, for the benefit of all such, that there is a much better way: namely--- to closely individualize, which is not always difficult; give the single remedy in potentized form, giving it time to act, and wait for reaction before repeating."

(Nash, Leaders in Homoeopathic Therapeutics P. 19)

(iii) "The merest tyro in prescribing could hardly mistake the symptoms of Pulsatilla for those of Nux vomica, and yet I have found physicians prescribing these remedies in alternation, at intervals of two or three hours."

(Nash, Leaders in Homoeopathic Therapeutics PP. 25-26)

Nash describes his purposes to offer this work to the profession as under:

First. — To fasten upon the mind of reader the strongest points in each remedy. Second. — To try to discourage the disposition to quarrel over Symptomatology and Pathology. Third. — To insist on to the fact that the question of dose is still an open one. Fourth. —To condemn the abuse of drugs both in old school and ours. Fifth. — To induce any old school physician, who would overcome prejudice so far as to read any or all of this book, to experiment along the lines I have indicated, believing that any such physician, of sound head and honest heart, will be irresistibly led to give Homoeopathy a large, and perhaps finally, the largest place in his confidence and practice.

(Nash, Leaders in Homoeopathic Therapeutics PP. 4-5)

Dr. S.M. Gunavante says about Nash's "Leaders",

"The first book we recommend for all beginners is the "Leaders in Homoeopathic Therapeutics" by Dr. E.B. Nash. This book provides an excellent introduction to Homoeopathy for beginners, covering philosophy, Materia Medica, therapeutics, potency, etc. with a "dose" of infectious enthusiasm as well. A dry subject is made very interesting as well as instructive. It repays repeated reading, and even veterans find it necessary to refer to it occasionally."

(Gunavante, Introduction to Homoeopathic Prescribing, P. 41)

Nash covers over 200 remedies, leading symptoms of each remedy in point form, followed by a friendly narrative drawing heavily on the author's own experience. This book gives some interesting insights into the thought process of one of the great old homoeopaths. Let us read a complete remedy from Nash's "Leaders in Homoeopathic Therapeutics" in order to know how skillfully this great teacher makes us learn use of our armamentarium in the fight against diseases.

NUX VOMICA

For very particular, careful, zealous persons, inclined to get excited or angry, spiteful, malicious disposition, mental workers or those having sedentary occupations.

Over-sensitiveness, easily offended; very little noise frightens, cannot bear the least even suitable medicine; faints easily from odors, etc.

Twitchings, spasms, convulsion, < slightest touch.

Chilliness, even during high fever; least uncovering brings on chilliness. Very red face.

Persons addicted to stimulants, narcotics, patent medicines, nostrums, debauchees, etc.

Frequent and ineffectual desire for stool or passes little at a time, > after stool.

Modalities: < uncovering, mental work, after eating, cold air, dry weather, stimulants, 9 A. M.; > wet weather, warm room, on covering, after stool.

Spasm (from simple twitchings to the clonic form); sensitiveness, nervous and chilliness are three general characteristics of this remedy.

Anxiety with irritability and inclination to commit suicide, but is afraid to die.

Sleepy in the evening, hours before bedtime; lies aware for an hour or two, at 3 or 4 A. M., then wants to sleep late in morning.

Awakens tired and weak and generally worse, with many complaints.

Stomach: Pressure an hour or two after eating as from a stone (immediately after, Kali bi., Nux m.).

Convulsions with consciousness (Strych.); < anger, emotion, touch, moving, alternate constipation and diarrhea (Ant. crud.).

Menses: Too early, profuse and lasting too long, with aggravation of all other complaints during their continuance.

Nux vomica acts better when given at night, during repose of mind and body; Sulph. in the morning.

* * * * *

Among the symptoms called characteristic, as given by Constantine Hering, are these:

"After aromatics in food or as medicine, particularly ginger, pepper, etc., and after almost any kind of so-called 'hot' medicines (Goullon)." Also, "will also benefit persons who have been drugged by mixtures, bitters, herbs and so-called vegetable pills, etc. -(B.)"

This is putting it in too wholesale a fashion. It would be true if said that Nux vomica will often benefit such cases. The fact is that it will benefit those cases in which the use of such drugs, aromatics, pills, etc. has brought about a condition that simulates the symptoms produced in the provings of Nux vomica, or in cases to which it is homoeopathic, and no others. Another fact is that things often do produce such a condition, and that is one reason why so many physicians are invariably prescribing Nux vomica the first thing, in cases coming from allopathic hands, without even examining the case, but it is unscientific. We have a law of cure and there are cases in which the Nux vomica condition is not present but another more similar remedy must be given. It does not alter the case to say, "Well, I did not know what had been given," for Nux vomica will neither antidote the effects of the drug poison nor cure the disease condition unless it is homoeopathically indicated, especially given in the dynamic form.

Here are two more of Hering's card symptoms, in which are given the temperaments that are most susceptible to the action of Nux:

"Oversensitiveness, every harmless word offends, every little noise frightens, anxious and beside themselves, they cannot bear the least even suitable medicines - (B)." And, "For very particular, careful, zealous persons, inclined to get excited and angry, or of a spiteful, malicious disposition."

This is a graphic picture of what is called the "Nervous temperament," and practice corroborates the truth of the value of these temperamatic indications for this remedy; but there are a number of remedies that have as markedly this so called nervous temperament, such as Chamomilla, Ignatia, Staphysagria, and others.

So no physician would be justified in prescribing Nux vomica on temperament alone, be the indication ever so clear. The whole case must come in. There seems to be another kind of condition belonging to this nervous group of Nux vomica that has not so much of excitability in it. "Hypochondriasis, with studious men, sitting too much at home, with abdominal complaints and costiveness."

Now if you take a second look at these cases, you will find that a very little irritation will arouse this kind out of their hypochondriac gloom and make them angry or irritable similar to the first condition, so that on the whole the first proves to be the predominant one.

If the gloomy or hypochondriac condition of mind persists, we will more likely have to look to such remedies as Aurum, Nat. mur. etc., to find the true similimum. These nervous symptoms of mind and body are wonderful leaders to the selection of the right remedy.

"Frequent and ineffectual desire to defecate or passing but small quantities of fæces at each attempt."

This symptom is pure gold. There are a few other remedies that have it, but none so positively and persistently.

It is the guiding symptom in the constipation to which Nux vomica is homoeopathic and in my experience will then, and then only, cure. Carroll Dunham wrote over twenty-five years ago on this symptom. He said, in effect -while Nux vomica or Bryonia are equal remedies for constipation there was never any reason for confounding them, or alternating them, as they were so different. The Nux vomica constipation was caused by irregular peristaltic action of the intestines, hence the frequent ineffectual desire; but the Bryonia constipation was caused by lack of secretion in the intestines. There was with Bryonia absolutely no desire, and the stools were dry and hard as if burnt.

And the above symptom is found not in constipation alone. It is always present in dysentry. The stools, though very frequently consisting of slimy mucus and blood, are very small and unsatisfactory. Dr.P.P. Wells pointed out the very reliable additional symptom for Nux vomica in dysentry -that the pains were very greatly relieved for a short time after every stool. This is not so with Mercury, but the pain and tenesmus continue after the stool, as it is sometimes well expressed as "a never-get-done" feeling. But it makes little difference whether the patient is afflicted with constipation, dysentery, diarrhoea or other diseases, if we have this frequent ineffectual desire for stool present we always think of Nux vomica first, and give it unless other symptoms contra-indicate it.

"Catamenia a few days before time, and rather too copious, or keeping on several days longer with complaints at the onset, which remain until after it is over."

This is also an oft-verified symptom of Nux vomica. Of course there are many other remedies for too early or too copious menstruation. Calcarea Ostrearum is not at all like Nux vomica. I have found that patients that required Nux vomica, for this condition could hardly ever take Pulsatilla for anything. For instance, if the patient had green, bland, thick discharge and you gave them Pulsatilla it would often bring down too early and profuse menses. In such cases I had to give Sepia which would act like a charm on the catarrh and not aggravate the menses.

These cases calling for Nux vomica. often occur in young girls or women at the climacteric. We often have the characteristic rectal troubles also present (Lilium tig.). The pains are pressing down and extend to the rectum and sometimes also to the neck of bladder. Inefficient labour pains, extending to the rectum, with desire for stool or frequent urination, are quickly relieved, and become efficient, after the administration of a dose of Nux vomica 200.

If, in addition, your menorrhagic patient is costive, has gastric troubles, and especially if generally < in the morning, we have an almost sure remedy in Nux vomica.

"Feels worse in the morning soon after awaking (Lach. and Nat. mur.), also after mental exertion (Nat carb., vertigo; Calc. ost., Sil., occipital); after eating (Anac. card., reverse) and in cold air (Puls., reverse)" If Bœnninghausen had never done anything but given us his incomparable chapter on aggravations and ameliorations, this alone would have immortalised him.

It seems to me, after profiting them in a practice of over thirty years, it is impossible to over estimate them. But some one will say perhaps -there are twenty-eight remedies in Allen's Bœnninghausen., in large caps, that are worse in the morning. That does not seem like coming very close to the choice of the remedy.

But when we look at those that are worse in the evening, we find thirty-eight remedies, and only eight of them occurring under both morning and evening, and these eight are worse not generally, but rather in some especial symptoms. For instance, in Rhus the loose cough is worse in the morning, the tight dry one in the evening.

So you see we are quite on the way to making a choice after all. But now take all the aggravations of Nux vomica as regards time, mind, gastric (symptoms), temperature etc., where can you find the combination so prominently under any remedy? Of course those physicians who are not able to appreciate anything but pathological symptoms have not much use for these modalities. But one thing is certain, they cannot do as good homœopathic work without as with them.

"Great heat, whole body burning hot, especially face red and hot, yet the patient cannot move or uncover in the least without feeling chilly." This condition of feverishness is of common occurrence and yields to Nux vomica with a promptness that would delight the heart of A. Lippe. It makes no difference what the name of the fever, whether inflammatory, remittent or fever accompanying sore throat, rheumatism, or any other local trouble, if we have these indications, we may confidently give this remedy and will not be often disappointed with the result. It took me years to learn the value of this symptom, because I was a routinist and thought that Aconite, Belladonna, or both in alteration, must be given in all cases where high fever was present. So I have some sympathy for young physicians now, who from false teachings have been led to the same error. But let me say here, for the benefit of all such, that there is a much better way: namely -to closely individualize, which is not always difficult; give the single remedy in the potentised form, giving it time to act, and wait for reaction before repeating.

Of course low potencies will often cure, and that in spite of alternation, over dosing and frequent repetition. But they will often fail, and in the great majority of cases will not accomplish anything like the satisfactory results of the true similimum, the single remedy and the single dose.

"After eating: (Kali bich, Nux moschata) sour taste pressure in the stomach an hour or two afterward, with hypochondriacal mood, pyrosis tightness about the waist; must loosen clothing (Lachesis, Calcarea, and Lycopodium), confused cannot use mind two or three hours after meal, epigastrium bloated, with pressure as from a stone in the stomach."

This is a group of symptoms as given in "Guiding Symptoms." There are so many symptoms given under the digestive organs that it shows that Nux vomica has really very wide range of action in gastric troubles. And there are no really characteristic and peculiar symptoms to mention, unless it be the peculiar aggravation of the stomach symptoms "an hour or two after eating," instead of immediately after as is the case with Nux moschata and Kali bichromicum. The pressure as from a stone occurs also in Bryonia and Pulsatilla.

More stress may be placed upon the cause of the stomach, liver and abdominal complaints for which Nux vomica is the remedy. For instance, coffee, alcoholic drinks, debauchery, abuse of drugs, business anxiety, sedentary habits, broken rest from long night watching (Cocc., Cup. met., Nit. ac.), too high living etc. So we find that Nux vomica is adapted to complaints arising from these causes, which is abundantly verified in practice.

One thing is very apt to be present in these cases: namely-the very characteristic rectal symptoms already noticed.

We ought not to leave Nux vomica without speaking of its great efficiency in headaches and backaches.

The headache often occurs in conjunction with gastric, hepatic, abdominal and hæmorrhoidal affections. Here also the modalities, more than the character of the pain, decide the choice. The aggravations are: from mental exertion, chagrin or anger; in open air (opposite Pulsatilla), on waking in the morning, after eating, from abuse of coffee or spirits, sour stomach, in the sunshine, on stooping, from light and noise, when moving or opening the eyes (Bryonia), from coughing high living or highly seasoned food, in stormy weather, after drugging, from masturbation, from constipation or haemorrhoids.

These headaches may or may not localize in any part of the head.

The patient is just as apt to say in one part of the head as another, and will often say, in no particular part, "it feels badly and aches all over."

The pains in the back are more peculiar. The patient is apt to have backache in bed, and must sit up to turn over; as turning or twisting the body, aggravates when standing (Sulphur) (worse when sitting, Kobalt, Pulsatilla, Rhus toxicod., Zincum) or sitting is especially painful. The pain is mostly located in the lumbar region, though it may be in the dorsa, and is often in connection (like Æsculus hipp.) with hæmmorhoids. Æsculus is especially < from walking or stooping. Backache caused by masturbation (Kobalt, < sitting; Staphysagria, lying at night) finds one of its best remedies in Nux vomica. We might here launch out into a description of the general action of Nux vomica upon the spinal cord, including the motor and sensory centers, etc. but that can all be found in other works. So now we will leave Nux, except as we refer to it in comparison while writing of other remedies. In reviewing of what we have written, we are impressed that some may be led to think that we have narrowed down the sphere of this truly great remedy too much. Let us say here, that it is not our aim in this work to write exhaustively upon any remedy, but to point out a few of the chief virtues and the characteristic symptoms, around which all the rest revolve.

To write exhaustively would be to write a complete materia medica.

In actual practice there are two kinds of cases that come to every physician. One is the case that may be prescribed for with great certainty of success on the symptoms that are styled characteristic and peculiar (Organon § 153.) The other is where in all the case there are no such symptoms appearing; then there is only one way, viz, to hunt for the remedy that, in its pathogenesis, contains what is called the "tout ensemble" of the case. The majority of the cases, however, do have, standing out like beacon lights. Some characteristic or keynote symptoms which guide to the study of the remedy that has the whole case in its pathogenesis.

HOMOEOPATHIC DRUG PICTURES

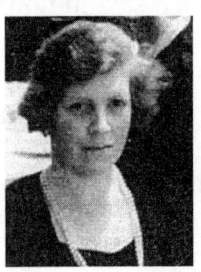

M.L. Tyler

Margaret Lucy Tyler (1857-1943) was a leading 19th century British Homoeopath. She was daughter of a homoeopath Sir H.J. Tyler. She was a protégé of Kent, though never studied with him. She worked in London Homoeopathic Hospital for over 40 years. With the money she inherited, she set up the Sir Henry James Tyler Scholarship Fund which sent several physicians, including Borland, and John Weir, to study with Kent. She authored,

1. Pointers to Common Remedies.
2. Acute Conditions, Injuries etc.
3. Homoeopathic Drug Pictures.
4. A Study of Kent's Repertory.
5. Different Ways of Finding Remedy.
6. Repertorizing.
7. Hahnemann's Conception of Chronic Diseases.
8. Homoeopathy, Introductory Lecture.

The early Materia Medicas contain unorganized collections of symptoms produced by drugs on healthy human beings. Although those Materia Medicas consist of purest effects of drugs ever known to mankind yet they do not contain such pictures of medicines as can easily be comprehended and matched to the pictures of diseases for homoeopathic purposes. Later, many of great homoeopaths compiled narrative Materia Medicas in which they organized symptoms and linked them to each other in order to sketch comprehensive and recognizable pictures of remedies. So Tyler's "Homoeopathic Drug Pictures" is one of those materia medicas (others being Kent's Lectures and Nash's Leaders etc.) which present coherent pictures of remedies. We can recognize remedies as living characters compare and contrast them to each other and match their pictures to the pictures of different totalities of symptoms.

Dr. Jugal Kishore, in his article "Introduction to Kent's Leactures" says,

"His (Kent) method of narrating drugs is popularly known as "Picture Method". His able and faithful student from Britain, Dr. Tyler, was another writer who gave us "drug pictures" of homeopathic remedies. It is no wonder that this book too has carved an important niche in our literature."

(Jugal Kishore, Introduction, Kent's Lectures P. 8)

Tyler's "Homoeopathic Drug Pictures" covers 125 remedies including some rares like Ornithogalum and Salicylic Acid. She commonly divides a remedy into two sections. The first section generally consists of quotes from pioneers of homoeopathy and great materia medica men like Hahnemann, Hering, Allen, Clarke, Hughes, Hale, Kent, Nash and Farrington etc. She tries not to miss any important point given by the pioneers. She emphasizes what has been emphasized by some or any of them. So by reading a remedy from Tyler's "Homoeopathic Drug Pictures" we learn many of its important points scattered in the work of many authorities of materia medica. She organizes symptoms and quotes in such a beautiful manner that a living picture of the remedy comes before the reader. She very skillfully justifies the title "Homoeopathic Drug Pictures".

She often starts a remedy by a beautiful interesting paragraph interlinking homoeopathic philosophy to the materia medica and the remedy under discussion,

"KALI BROMATUM... "Bromides"--- practically always "Pot brom." that powerful inhibiter, that grand suppresser, in almost universal use for the treatment of epilepsy, sleeplessness, "nerves", and yet which, as commonly administered, has never cured the chronic conditions for which it is prescribed, and never can.

How do we know this? Simply by the fact that the dose has to be always increased, as through the months or years the patient gradually asserts himself, and gets the better of the drug. You see there are two ways of prescribing. You may give a drug in order to do something to a patient, to "depress his nervous system and more or less paralyze the higher functions of his brain"; but this does not recommend itself as an ideal form of treatment to the homoeopath, whose concern is, always, the vital stimulation of the patient, according to definite laws, whereby he is roused to cure himself. Drugs do not cure, popular opinion notwithstanding. Cure must come from within; or there is no cure."

(M.L. Tyler, Homoeopathic Drug Pictures, P. 462)

"LACHESIS... The greater the poison the greater the remedy; and some of the most rapidly-acting and heroic medicines in desperate diseases are the snake poisons. They cure, of course, just the conditions they produce: but, when used for healing purposes, these poisons must be given in small, innocuous doses; and only to persons whose symptoms (physical, mental or moral) resemble the poison symptoms. . Where this is the case, the curative power is amazing."

(M.L. Tyler, Homoeopathic Drug Pictures, P. 492)

While first section of a remedy is a summary of many materia medicas, the second section, which consists of important symptoms in point form, is précis of all the above discussion. She names them "Black Letter Symptoms". She often gives example cases cured by the remedy under discussion which generate a practicle picture of the remedy in mind of the reader. She also compares remedies very finely and enables the reader confidently select a remedy over others. Her style is narrative and flowing which makes it a must readable and great book for the neophyte.

ARGENTUM NITRICUM

Drugs elicit queer and characteristic symptoms, mental and physical, from their provings: and when these match the queer and characteristic symptoms, mental and physical, of sick persons, they cure. The nearer the correspondence the more certain the cure.

Argentum nitricum—silver nitrate—is the "devil's stone" or "hell stone" of Old School which has not much use of it, except as Lunar Caustic: because in allopathic doses, or when accidentally swallowed during the process of cauterizing the throat, it has turned people permanently blue—a condition known as " argyria." With us it is most precious remedy, and no other can take its place.

The earlier provings of Argentum nitricum given in Allen's Encyclopedia are, as we shall see, chiefly concerned with its physical symptoms, which are very definite and suggestive, and have led to splendid curative work in stomach conditions, etc. but other provings, given in Hering's Guiding Symptoms, bring out its interesting and unique mental peculiarities; and these are our most precious indications for its use.

Remedies, as we Homeopaths learn to realize them, step forth as personalities. They haunt us in 'bus and tram, and confront us in our patients. They become of temperaments—mental and physical. They have likes and dislikes, cravings and aversions: sensitiveness to meteoric conditions, as well as to human intercourse and environment. We realize their terrors, real or imaginary—their strange obsessions. And in measure as this is so; we are able to apply them with success for the relief of persons of like idiosyncrasies and distresses.

Silver nitrate is a remedy of very vivid personality, quite unlike all others. It has such strange weaknesses and self-tormentings! —and known it so well, and having experienced its splendid power to help, it may seem a strange thing to say, but one regards it with something like affection.

Old School has no conception of the wonderful power to strengthen and to comfort, of this remedy. Its mental and intellectual distresses are great.

Let KENT, in his vivid way, detail for us some of the mental inwardness of Arg Nit. which we must condense. He describes "disturbances in memory—disturbances in reason." He says Arg nit is irrational: does strange things, and comes to strange conclusions: does foolish things.

"He is tormented by the inflowing of troublesome thoughts, which torment him till he is in a hurry and fidget, and he goes out and walks and walks, and the faster he walks the faster he thinks he must walk, and he walks till fatigued, he has an impulse that he is going to have I fit—or he is going to a sickness. A strange thought comes to his mind that if he goes past a certain corner of the street he will create a sensation—perhaps fall down in fit: and to avoid that he will go round the block. He avoid going round that corner, for fear he will do something strange.

"There is an inflowing of thoughts into his mind. In crossing a bridge, or high place—the thought that he might kill himself—or jump off, or what if he should jump off: and sometimes the actual impulse to jump off that bridge into the water. When looking out of a high window, the thought comes into his head, what an awful thing would be to jump out of that window; and sometimes the impulse comes to actually jump out.

"There is a fear of death—the over-anxious state that death is near (Aconit). When looking forward to something he has to do, or has promised to do, or in expectation of things, he is anxious. When about to meet an engagement, he is anxious. Breaks into a sweat with anxiety . . . when going to wedding—

to the opera—to church, the anxiety is attended with fear—even to diarrhoea (Gels).

"So we have a wonderful queer medicine.

"Mental exhaustion, headaches, nervous excitement and trembling, and organic troubles of heart and liver; in business men, students, brain workers, in those subject to long excitement, in actors who have kept up a long time the excitement of appearing well in public.....

"Like Pulsatilla, Arg nit wants cold air, cold drinks. Suffocates in warm room. Cannot go to church or opera, must stay at home. Dreads a crowd, dreads certain places.

"And then the physical side . . .. Full of ulcerations especially on internal parts, and mucous membranes. Kent says this tendency to ulcerate seems rather strange; peculiar that it should have in its pathogenesis such a tendency, when the Old School has been using it to cauterize ulcers, and yet it heals them up..... It has cured prolonged and almost inveterate ulceration of stomach, when there has been vomiting of blood.

"Do not forget that this medicine is one of the most flatulent medicines in the books. He is distended to bursting; gets scarcely relief from passing flatus or eructations.

"Desire sugar: feels he must have it and it makes him sick. So marked is the aggravation from sugar that the nursing infant will get a green diarrhoea if the mother eats candy". Kent gives a case where nothing helped the baby "till he found out that the mother ate candy—her husband brought her home a pound of candy every day. The baby did not get well till it got Arg nit and the mother stopped eating candy.

Arg nit has the most intense eye symptoms: catarrhal, ulcerative; to opacities of cornea. But all worse for heat and relieved by cold. Profuse purulent discharge from lids".

NASH quotes Allen and Norton in regard to eyes, "The greatest service that Argentum nitricum performs is in purulent ophthalmia. With a large experience in both hospital and private practice, we have not lost a single eye from this disease, and every one has been treated with internal remedies, most of them with Argentum nitricum of a high potency, 30th or 200th. We have witnessed the most intense chemosis, with strangulated vessels, most profuse purulent discharge, even the cornea beginning to get hazy and looking as though it would slough, subside rapidly under Argentum nitricum internally. The subjective symptoms are almost none. Their very absence, with the profuse purulent discharge, and the swollen lids from the collection of pus in the eye, or swelling of the sub-conjunctival tissue of the lids themselves, indicate the drug." (One may say that such a case, in a child, during the 1914-18 War, with Arg nit 200 and bathing the eye with normal saline, was amazingly better the next day, and soon well. This was impressed on one's memory, since eye cases have seldom come one's way.)

Arg nit has some peculiar physical symptoms: Sick in the throat sensation (Hepar etc), simultaneous vomiting and purging—gushing both ways" like Arsenicum.

All these things Argentum nitricum has caused and can (and has) cured.

Now for more of physical symptoms, extracted from Allen's Encyclopedia.

"Anxiety which makes him walk rapidly.

Vertigo.

Vertigo, general debility of limbs and trembling.

Headache relieved by binding something tightly round head.

Ophthalmia: better cool open air, intolerable in warm room.

Ophthalmia with intense pains.

Grey spots and bodies in shape of serpents move before vision.

The canthi are red as blood: the caruncula lachrimalis is swollen, Stands out of the corner of the eye like a lump of red flesh: clusters of intensely red vessels extend from the inner canthus to the cornea.

The conjunctiva is puckered and interstitially distended. Vanishing of sight. Must constantly wipe off the mucus which obstructs vision.

Sickly appearance. Appearance of old age.

Pain in teeth: worse when chewing—eating sour things—cold things.

Painful red tip of tongue.

Rawness throat. Rawness and soreness.

Thick tenacious mucus in throat.

Sensation as if splinter were lodged in throat when swallowing.

Uvula and fauces dark red.

Irresistible desire for sugar.

Violent belching.

Nausea after eating.

Constant nausea, and frequent efforts to vomit.

Vomiting and diarrhoea with violent colicky pains.

Desire to vomit, with sensation as if head were in a vice.

Violent cardialgia.

After yawning, sensation as if stomach would burst. Wind presses upwards.

Painful swelling in pit of stomach with great anxiety.

Abdomen swollen and distended, with much flatulence.

A slight colic wakes him from uneasy slumber, and has sixteen evacuations of greenish, very foetid mucus, with a quantity of noisy flatus.

Four evacuations of green mucus, with retching, vomiting of mucus.

(After having eaten sugar greedily in the evening, he was attacked with) scanty watery diarrhoea about midnight, accompanied with flatulent colic, and much noisy flatulence during the evacuation.

Violent diarrhoea, like spinach flacks.

Palpitation and irregular action of heart.

Staggering and paralytic heaviness of lower limbs.

Rigidity in calves: great debility and weariness in calves, can scarcely walk.

Tremulous weakness. Trembling and tremulous sensation.

Convulsions.

Peculiar discoloration of skin, from grey-blue, violet or bronze-coloured tinges to the real black.

Skin brown, tense, hard",

As said, Arg nit is one of the great remedies for the terrors of anticipation. It has Examination funk. Its nervousness in anticipation of a coming ordeal will go as far as diarrhoea — (Gelsemium). One of doctors makes great play with his "Funk Pills" — Arg nit. The anticipation remedies are rather scattered through Kent's repertory, but we have colleted the following, which should be interested as a rubric.

ARG NIT, Ars, Carbo veg, GELS, Lyco, Med, Pb, Phos-a, Sil.

Arg nit has also claustrophobia. Wants the end seat in pew: to be near the door in church or theatre: needs an easy escape. "Even in the streets the sight of high houses always made him giddy and caused him to stagger: it seemed as if the houses on both sides would approach and crush him." Arg nit cannot look — and cannot look up.

Here are some cured symptoms . . . . . . "When walking becomes faint with anxiety, which makes him walk faster". . . . . "Often wakes his wife or child, to have someone to talk to" . . . . . 'Fears to be alone, because he thinks he will die." . . . . . . "When walking, fears he will have a fit, or die, which makes him walk faster," . . . . "Distressing idea, that all his undertakings must and would fail." . . . . . "Does not work, thinking it will do him harm, or that he is not able to stand It." . . . . . "Fears, if passing a certain corner or building that he will drop down and create a sensation; is relieved by going in another direction . ...

* * *

A poor little schoolgirl of six, in such terrors of anticipating that, when the school bell rang, she put her head in her hands, and vomited. Argentum nit finished that trouble promptly and entirely, and sent her rapidly to school, to do well there.

A weak boy of 4 was curiously ill—mentally. The history was: Measles before he was two: then double pneumonia and (?) meningitis. He "rolled his head" and had evidently marked opisthotonos ("was bent like a bow, backwards, between head and heels"). "When he began to walk, walked backwards". Now had "terrible nights, with much screaming" and "mad" attacks by day. . Was in terror of his father, by night—" Daddy might look at me!". He said of people, "They make me bleed and I'll make them bleed". He said the next house was "going to fall on him"; that "the clouds were coming down on him". Great fear of noise.

The first medicine did not help much. But after a couple of doses of Arg nit the next report was, "Very much better. Lost the things coming down on him. Fears all gone." Later he needed a few doses of Belladonna, and then its "chronic" Calcarea; and in a few months he was well and normal. But for a weak boy to put up such a plea for Argentum nitricum, by such very peculiar and characteristic symptoms, was curious.

Homoeopathy can do wonderful things in making children happy and normal.

A youthful dyspeptic, with almost daily severe flatulence and bursting sensation, worse for afternoon tea and long into the night, relieved pro tem by either Pulsatilla or Carbo veg, but always recurring, took Arg nit in potency. Result, the gastric symptoms ceased to trouble, in fact, never again did trouble the same extent. Puls and Carb v had been palliative only—Arg nit had proved curative.

But the Arg nit having proved such a boon was continued for some time, till a new, most distressing symptom appeared—numbness in the forearms at night. The wristbands of the nightdress had to be cut, everything pulled from arms; nothing must touch or press them. This was only a proving of Argentum nitricum and when this discontinued was soon forgotten, never recur . . . . . Since when, when patients have, from time to time, complained of such numbness in the arms at night, Arg nit has cured them.

The symptom is found is Clarke's Dictionary. He says "In a proving by myself, one of the most marked symptoms was a kind of numb sensitiveness of the skin of arms—a hyperaesthetic—anaesthetic state; increased sensitiveness to touch, but diminished power of distinguishing sensation."

Symptoms group often lead one to a particular remedy. Desire for sweets, desire for salt, can't stand heat, makes one think of Argentum nitricum. And if you find the patient cannot look down from a height, you may be sure. No other remedy has just that symptom complex.

One may note here that Dr.Clarke's remedy for Examination funk was Aethusa cynapium, "fool's parsley"—well named! One of its characteristic symptoms is "Inability to think, or fix the attention." He says "guided by this symptom I gave it an undergraduate preparing for examination, with complete success. He had been compelled to give up studies, but was able to resume them, and passed a brilliant examination. To little waif in an orphan home who suffered from severe headaches and inability to fix his attention on his lessons, I sent a single dose of Aethusa, at rare intervals with very great relief. The little boy asked for the medicine himself subsequently on a return of the old symptoms."

With Argentum nit the condition is apprehension—ill with anxiety in regard to what is before him: --fear of future. With Aethusa, it is simply inability to fix the attention, or to think.

Homoeopathy is very definite: and one remedy, even if you label both "funk pill", will not do for the other!

LECTURES ON MATERIA MEDICA
By J.T. Kent

&

COMPARATIVE STUDY ON KENT'S MATRIA MEDICA
By A.Gaskin

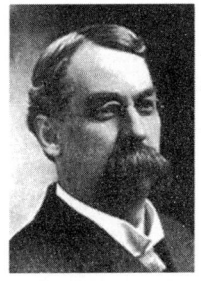

J.T. Kent

Kent is one of our great masters. He is one of those pioneers without any of them homoeopathy of the day is incomplete. One would be justified to say that Hahnemann presented homoeopathy to the world whereas Kent explained it and made it understood. There would be hardly a classical homoeopath in the world that would have not studied and utilized Kent's writings. At present, when you are reading this book there would be hundreds of homoeopaths in the world studying Kent's writings.

Kent was born on 31, March1849 in Woodhull, New York. He worked as professor of Materia Medica at St. Louis Homoeopathic Medical College, professor of Materia Medica and dean of the Post Graduate School of Homoeopathy Philadelphia, professor of Materia Medica in Hahnemann Medical College and Hospital Chicago and Hering Medical College and Hospital. He founded Post Graduate School in Philadelphia. He became president of the International

Hahnemannian Association (IHA) in 1887. He died on 6 June 1916 leaving his immortal work for posterity in the form of following books.
1. Repertory of the Homoeopathic Materia Medica.
2. Lectures on Homoeopathic Materia Medica.
3. Lectures on Homoeopathic Philosophy.
4. Lesser Writings, New Remedies, Clinical cases.
5. What The Doctor Needs To Know In Order To Make A Successful Prescription.

Dr. Jugal Kishore narrates the interesting story of Kent's conversion to Homoeopathy as follows,

"Like Hering and some of the great men of homoeopathy, Kent was converted to homoeopathy in spite of himself. His first wife was seriously ill. No amount of eclectic and allopathic treatment could help her. She entreated her husband to seek medicinal advice and help from a known homoeopath in their neighbourhood. To satisfy her whim he called Dr. Phelan, the homoeopath. He watched him, with possibly contemptuous amusement, taking the case-history and later his giving her some globules to be dissolved in water and taken according to his directions until she fell asleep. Mrs. Kent had been suffering from sleeplessness for days and nothing had helped her the least in giving her sleep. Kent chuckled within himself when Dr. Phelan mentioned about her getting sleep from the medicated water. He, however, fulfilled his part of the contract by giving her the first dose. The second dose to be given to her was delayed because Dr. Kent became absorbed in his books. When he remembered about the dose, he found her fast asleep. This was the first time that she had fallen into such a natural and sound sleep. This incident started his thinking. Under the care of Dr. Phelan, Mrs. Kent made a steady progress from the next day onwards. This was enough for Kent to throw himself heart and soul into the study of homoeopathic science."

(Jugal Kishore, "Introduction", Kent's Lectures, P. 9)

Kent was very intelligent and was blessed by the Creator with great creative qualities. He studied homoeopathy with thorough concentration and soon became aware of its real soul. Now he started teaching Homoeopathic Materia Medica in Homoeopathic colleges and for this teaching he needed to study Dr. Hering's "The Guiding Symptoms of Our Materia Medica". We know this is a big book that consists of 10 volumes and covers nearly all proved remedies. For Kent also it was too big to retain in the mind. While studying this book Kent brought into use his great creative qualities and remedies seemed to him like living characters. So in his "Lectures on Homoeopathic Materia Medica" he sketched living pictures of remedies by comparing, contrasting, analyzing, synthesizing and interlinking their symptoms. These descriptive pictures leave long lasting impressions on mind of the reader.

In medical history Kent is notable for denying the conventional germ-theory of infectious diseases. He says in his "Lesser Writings",

"Most doctors have gone crazy over the 'vicious microbes' as being the cause of disease, and think that the little fellows are exceedingly dangerous"

"As a matter of fact, the microbes are scavengers. I wonder if scientists reflect when they make statements about bacteria. Naturally they would say that the more bacteria the more danger, but this is not so. It is well known that shortly after death a prick from a scalpel is a serious matter. This is due to ptomaine of the corpse; but when the cadaver has become green and filled with bacteria it is comparatively harmless."

(J.T. Kent, Lesser Writings, P. 663)

He further says,

"The microbe is not the cause of disease. We should not be carried away by these idle Allopathic dreams and vain imaginations but should correct the vital force".

"Save the life of the patient first and don't worry about the bacteria. They are useless things".

The bacterium is an innocent feller, and if he carries disease he carries the Simple Substance which causes disease, jus as an elephant would".

(J.T. Kent, Lesser Writings, P. 663)

"The man who believes that he is directing his remedies against germs, against worms or against a tumor the patient may have, is in extreme darkness, if he cannot perceive that a healthy man will have healthy tissues, healthy blood, and therefore there can be no soil for germs, worms or morbid growths".

(J.T. Kent, Lesser Writings, P. 204)

In homoeopathy Kent is respected for his marvelous work for the profession. His repertory is an indispensable tool of practice for every classical homoeopath. One who studies and understands his "Lectures on Homoeopathic Philosophy" and "Lectures on Homoeopathic Materia Medica" becomes a sound homoeopath.

Kent's "Lectures on Homoeopathic Materia Medica" is a well know classical homoeopathy book. It bears many qualities for which its importance and use has not been decreased even after a whole century. Some of its salient features are as under:

Kent interlinks Materia Medica with philosophy and teaches the reader how to use homoeopathic remedies according to the principles of homoeopathy. His "Lectures" are full of philosophical admonitions. While giving a therapeutic hint he always says, "If the symptoms agree", "when the symptoms agree",

"It (Lycopodium) is also suitable in girls at puberty when the time for the first menstrual flow to appear has come, but it does not come. She goes on to 15, 16, 17 or 18 without development, the breasts do not enlarge, and the ovaries do not perform their function. When the symptoms agree Lyco. establishes the reaction, the breasts begin to grow, the womanly bearing begins to come, and the child becomes a woman".

(J.T. Kent, Lectures on Materia Medica, P. 712)

(Pulsatilla) "Nux-vomica has a free, easy breathing in open air, but when he goes into the warm room his nose stuffs up, which also occurs at night, though the water drips on the pillow yet he stuffs up like Puls., Bry., and the Iodine preparations, Iodide of Arsenic and Cyclamen. Do not understand me to have given remedies for hay fever; we cannot lay down remedies for diseases. The whole constitution must be most carefully examined."

(J.T. Kent, Lectures on Materia Medica, P. 864)

"The Silica cough is a dangerous one; the remedy suits the early stage of phthisis; when the lung is not extensively involved; it suits a cough of catarrhal character when the symptoms agree."

(J.T. Kent, Lectures on Materia Medica, P. 934)

"We pass now to the female genitalia, which form a center for a great deal of trouble in the remedy. A routine saying about Actea is that it makes confinement easy. That is not a legitimate saying concerning any remedy and such expressions encourage routine practice. It is true that when this remedy has been given to pregnant women in accordance with its symptoms it has proved capable of making confinement easy. But the way it has been given has been the routine practice of giving it in the tincture or in the 2d or 3d, until the patient was under its influence even when it was not indicated, as it was not similar to the case. But the homoeopathic physician never practices in this way. A remedy fits a general condition when the symptoms of that general condition are found in the remedy. Remember that it does so because all the symptoms agree. "Pain in the uterine region, darting from side to side. Bearing down and pressing out." These bearing down sensations, taken with all the other states that relate to the patient in general, show that it is a very useful remedy in prolapsus of the uterus. It has the relaxation of the parts. Do not suppose that our remedies are not sufficient to cure these conditions, when the symptoms agree. It is true that remedies will cure prolapsus when the symptoms agree, and at no other time. If it fits the patient in general, these bearing down sensations will go away, the patient will be made comfortable, and an examination will finally show that the parts are in normal condition. You cannot prescribe for the prolapsus; you must prescribe for the woman. You cannot prescribe for one symptom, because there are probably fifty remedies that have that symptom."

(J.T. Kent, Lectures on Materia Medica, P. 33)

In this way Kent emphasizes to base the selection of medicine on the totality of symptoms which is the soul of Homoeopathic Science. His followers are the strict followers of the principles.

Kent draws, as said before, living and dynamic pictures of remedies which are engraved in the mind of the reader. Dr. Jugal Kishore says,

"Right from Hahnemann onwards, the records of provings prepared in schematic form were presented as Materia Medica. Before Kent, the best writers and teachers of materia medica were Hering, Dunham and Farrington. The materia medica was presented as a list of symptoms arranged according to Hahnemann's schema. It was obvious that it was not possible to memorize the symptoms. Kent held that materia medica can be learned and not memorized. Of course it required a careful and diligent study. His emphasis was on understanding of each remedy in its entirety and not on memorizing of unrelated symptoms.

(Jugal Kishore, "Introduction", Kent's Lectures, P.3)

Kent was the first to see clearly how to present our materia medica to the beginners; how to lay down precise guidelines regarding the hierarchy of evaluation of different kinds of symptoms.

(Jugal Kishore, "Introduction", Kent's Lectures, P.5)

Let us read a part of Carbo Veg from Kent's "Lectures on Homoeopathic Materia Medica" and see how skillfully and beautifully he personifies a remedy,

"We will take up the study of Vegetable Charcoal - Carbo Veg. It is a comparatively inert substance made medicinal and powerful, and converted into a great healing agent, by grinding it fine enough. By dividing it sufficiently, it becomes similar to the nature of sickness and cures folks. The Old School use it in tablespoonful doses to correct acidity of the stomach. But it is a great monument to Hahnemann. It is quite inert in crude form and the true healing powers are not brought out until it is sufficiently potentized. It is one of those deep acting, long-acting antipsoric medicines. It enters deeply into the life, in its proving it develops symptoms that last a long time, and it cures conditions that are of long standing-those that come on slowly and insidiously. It affects the vascular system especially; more particularly the venous side of the economy, the heart, and the whole venous System. Sluggishness is a good word to think of when examining the pathogenesis of Carbo Veg. Sluggishness, laziness, turgescence, these are words that will come into your mind frequently, because these states occur so frequently in the symptomatology. Everything about the economy is sluggish, turgid, distended and swollen. The hands are puffed; the veins are puffed; the body feels full and turgid; the head feels full, as if full of blood. The limbs feel dull, so that the patient wants to elevate the feet to let the blood run out. The veins are lazy, relaxed and paralyzed. Vaso-motor paralysis. The veins of the body are enlarged; the extremities have varicose veins.

The whole mental state, like the physical, is slow. The mental operations are slow. Slow to think; sluggish; stupid; lazy. Cannot whip himself into activity, or rouse a desire to do anything. Wants to lie down and doze. The limbs are clumsy; they feel enlarged. The skin is dusky. The capillary circulation is engorged. The face is purple. Any little stimulating food or drink will bring a flush to that dusky face. When you see people gather round a table where wine is served you can pick out the Carbo Veg. patients, because their faces will be flushed; in a little while it passes off and they get purple again dusky - almost a dirty duskiness. The skin is lazy; sluggish."

(J.T. Kent, Lectures on Materia Medica, PP. 370-71)

Although Kent's "Lectures" is a great study book yet it is not a full Materia Medica. For full and detailed knowledge of symptoms we would need to refer to original materia medica books and repertory. Dr. Jugal Kishore says,

"Although Kent's novel method of presenting materia medica was found to be very effective, he himself advised the students not to depend entirely on the drug pictures. They must go back to larger textbooks giving the symptoms of the drugs. More than that they must go to the repertories also for constant reference and comparative study. The materia medica and repertory go hand in hand and nobody can master either of the subjects without referring to other. It has been found that great repertorians were also the masters of materia medica. Of course no repertory can be made or improved without constant study of our materia medicas. It is a hard a laborious study but the rewards are none the less as sweets".

(Jugal Kishore, "Introduction", Kent's Lectures, PP.8-9)

Another marvelous attribute of Kent's "Lectures" is its valuable comparisons by which he makes the reader learn individualization of remedies. Thus he teaches us how to differentiate and individualize remedies by comparing them and enables us to pick out the most similar one. He not only compares remedies but also clearly and forcefully warns against misuse of one in place of another. One can hardly make such mistakes after having read Kent's "Lectures",

"It (Calc-c) has burning in the vertex, and this is often present with coldness of the forehead, or the whole head may feel cold, except a burning spot on the vertex. Calcarea will again have cold head and icy cold feet when walking in cold air, or in very cold weather; but as soon as the feet get warm they go to the other extreme, and burn so that he puts them out of bed. This has often led inexperienced prescribers to prescribe Sulph. because that is a keynote of Sulph. All keynote prescribers give Sulph. whenever the patient puts the feet out of bed, but a number of remedies have burning feet, hot feet, so we are not limited to Sulph."

(J.T. Kent, Lectures on Materia Medica, P. 321)

(Chamomilla) "Burning of the soles at night; puts the feet out of bed. All the routine prescribers whenever the patient is known to put the feet out of bed give Sulph, yet there is a large list of remedies with hot feet, burning soles, and all of them will put the feet out of bed, of course, to cool them off. There is no reason they should all get Sulphur."

(J.T. Kent, Lectures on Materia Medica, P. 423)

A. Gaskin, a contemporary British homoeopath, has collected all comparisons from Kent's "Lectures" and made a new book very useful for beginners. He has arranged all comparisons of Kent in a systematic way. So this book tells us which remedies can be compared to one and another and what is the difference in them in spite of some resembling symptomatology. Let us read a remedy, Carbo-Veg, from Kent's LECTURES ON MATERIA MEDICA and then its comparisons from A. Gaskin's "Comparative Study on Kent's Materia Medica".

CARBO VEGETABILIS

We will take up the study of Vegetable Charcoal - Carbo veg. It is a comparatively inert substance made medicinal and powerful, and converted into a great healing agent, by grinding it fine enough. By dividing it sufficiently, it becomes similar to the nature of sickness and cures folks. The Old School use it in tablespoonful doses to correct acidity of the stomach. But it is a great monument to Hahnemann. It is quite inert in crude form and the true healing powers are not brought out until it is sufficiently potentized. It is one of those deep acting, long-acting antipsoric medicines. It enters deeply into the life, in its proving it develops symptoms that last a long time, and it cures conditions that are of long standing-those that come on slowly and insidiously. It affects the vascular system especially; more particularly the venous side of the economy, the heart, and the whole venous System. Sluggishness is a good word to think of when examining the pathogenesis of Carbo veg. Sluggishness, laziness, turgescence, these are words that will come into your mind frequently, because these, states occur so frequently in the symptomatology. Everything about the economy is sluggish, turgid, distended and swollen. The hands are puffed; the veins are puffed; the body feels full and turgid; the head feels full, as if full of blood. The limbs feel dull, so that the patient wants to elevate the feet to let the blood run out. The veins are lazy, relaxed and paralyzed. Vaso-motor paralysis. The veins of the body are enlarged; the extremities have varicose veins.

The whole mental state, like the physical, is slow. The mental operations are slow. Slow to think; sluggish; stupid; lazy. Cannot whip himself into activity, or rouse a desire to do anything. Wants to lie down and doze. The limbs are clumsy; they feel enlarged. The skin is dusky. The capillary circulation is engorged. The face is purple. Any little stimulating food or drink will bring a flush to that dusky face. When you see people gather round a table where wine is served you can pick out the Carbo veg. patients, because their faces will be flushed; in a little while it passes off and they get purple again dusky - almost a dirty duskiness. The skin is lazy; sluggish.

Running through the remedy there is burning. Burning in the veins, burning in the capillaries, burning in the head, itching and burning of the skin. Burning in inflamed parts. Internal burning and external coldness. Coldness, with feeble circulation, with feeble heart. Icy coldness. Hands and feet cold and dry, or cold and moist. Knees cold; nose cold; ears cold; tongue cold. Coldness in the stomach with burning.

Fainting. Covered all over with a cold sweat, as in collapse. Collapse with cold breath, cold tongue, cold face. Looks like a cadaver. In all these conditions of coldness the patient wants to be fanned.

Bleeding runs all through the remedy. Oozing of blood from inflamed surfaces. Black bleeding from ulcers. Bleeding from the lungs; from the uterus; from the bladder. Vomiting of blood. Passive haemorrhage. On account of the feeble circulation a capillary oozing will start up and continue. The remedy hardly ever has what may be called an active gushing flow, such as belongs to Belladonna, Ipecac, Aconite, Secale, and such remedies, where the flow comes with violence; but it is a passive capillary oozing. The women suffer from this kind of bleeding; a little blood oozing all the time, so that the menstrual period is prolonged. Oozing of blood after confinement, that ought to be stopped immediately by contractions. There are no contractions of the blood vessels; they are relaxed. Black venous oozing. After a surgical operation there is no contraction and retraction of the blood vessels. An injury to the skin bleeds easily. The arteries have all been tied and closed, but the little veins do not seem to have any contractility in their walls. An inflamed part may bleed. Feeble heart; relaxed veins.

Again, ulceration. If you have a case, such as I have described, with relaxation of the blood vessels and feebleness of the tissues, you need not be surprised if there is no repair, no tissue making. So, when a part is injured, it will slough. If an ulcer is once established, it will not heal. The tissues are indolent. Hence we have indolent ulcers; body, ichorous, acrid, thin discharges from ulcers. The skin ulcerates; the mucous membranes ulcerate. Ulcers in the mouth and in the throat. Ulceration everywhere because of that relaxed and feeble condition. Poor tissue making, or none at all, "The blood stagnates in the capillaries," is the way it reads in the text.

You can see how easy it would be for these feeble parts to develop gangrene. Any little inflammation or congestion becomes black or purple and sloughs easily that is all that is necessary to make gangrene. It is a wonderful remedy in septic conditions-blood poisoning, especially after surgical operations and after shock. It is a useful remedy in septic conditions; in scarlet fever; in any disease which takes on a sluggish form, with purplish and mottled appearance of the skin. In Carbo veg. the sleep is so full of anxiety that it may be said to be awful. On going to sleep there is anxiety, suffering, jerking, twitching, and he has the horrors. Everything is horrible. Horrible visions; sees ghosts. A peculiar sluggish, death-like sleep, with visions. The Carbo veg. patient wakens in anxiety and covered with cold sweat. Exhaustion. Unrefreshed after sleep. And thus the whole patient is prostrated by his sleep. So anxious that he does not want to go to sleep. Anxiety in the dark. Anxiety with dyspnoea as if he would suffocate. Anxiety so great that he can not lie down.

In Carbo veg. indifference is a very prominent symptom. Inability to perceive or to feel the impressions that circumstances ought to arouse. His affections are practically blotted out, so that nothing that is told him seems to arouse or disturb him. "Heard everything without feeling pleasantly or unpleasantly, and without thinking about it." Horrible things do not seem to affect him much; pleasant things do not affect him. He does not quite know whether he loves his wife and children or not. This is a part of the sluggishness, the inability to think or meditate, all of which is due to the turgescence. Sluggishness of the veins. Head feels full; distended. His mind is in confusion and he cannot think. He cannot bring himself to realize whether a thing be so or not, or whether he loves his family or not, or whether he hates his enemies or not. Benumbed stupid. There is another state--- anxiety and nightly fear of ghosts, anxiety as if possessed; anxiety on closing the eyes; anxiety lying down in the evening; anxiety again on waking. He is easily frightened. Starting and twitching on going too sleep.

The headaches are mostly occipital. His whole head is turgid, full, distended. He feels as if the scalp was too tight. Everything is bound up in the head. Awful occipital headaches. Cannot move, cannot turn over, cannot lie on the side, cannot be jarred, because it, seems as if the head would burst, as if something was grasping the occiput. Dull headache in the occiput. Violent pressive pain in the lower portion of the occiput. Head feels heavy. When the pain is in the occiput the head feels drawn back to the pillow, or as if it could not be lifted from the pillow. Like Opium; he cannot lift the head from the pillow. Painful throbbing in the head during inspiration. The Carbo veg. patient takes short breaths, quietly, keeping just as still as possible, until finally he is compelled to take a deep breath, and it comes out with a sharp moan. Headache as from contraction of the scalp. Painful stitches through the whole head when coughing; the whole head burns. Intense heat of the head; burning pain. Rush of the blood to the head followed by nose-bleed. Congestion to the head with spasmodic constriction, nausea, and pressure over the eyes. A feeling as of an oncoming coryza from an overheated room. Many of these headaches come on from taking cold, from coryza, from slacking up of an old catarrh. The Carbo veg. patient suffers from chronic catarrh. He is at his best when he has a free discharge from the nose, but if he takes cold and the discharge stops congestion to the head comes. He cannot stand suppression of discharges. Headaches come on every time he takes cold; from cold damp weather; from going into a cold damp place and becoming chilled. Awful occipital headache, or headache over the eyes, or headache involving the whole head, with pounding like hammers. These states are like Kali bichromicum, Kali iodatum and Sepia. Many of these headaches are due to stopped catarrhal conditions.

The hair falls out by the handful. Eruptions come out upon the head. School girls and boys, too, who are sluggish, slow to learn, and suffer from night terrors; they will not sleep alone, or go into a dark room without someone with them. They have headaches, worse from pressure of the hat. A long time after taking off the hat they still feel the pressure. Sweat, cold sweat; particularly sweat of the head and of the forehead. The Carbo veg. patient breaks out into a copious sweat, appearing first on the forehead, and the sweat is cold. The forehead feels cold to the hand, and any wind blowing upon it will produce pain; he wants it covered up. Head sensitive to cold. If he becomes overheated and like head perspires, and then a draft strikes that sweating head, his catarrh will stop at once and headaches will come on. His knees and hands and feet get cold, and he sweats without relief.

The eye symptoms are troublesome, and they often occur along with the headache. Burning pain in the eyes. The eyes become lustreless, deep-set, and the pupils do not react to light. He feels sluggish mentally, and does not want to think. He wants to sit or lie around, for every exertion gives him a headache. Whenever this state is present the eyes show it. You know he is sick because the bright, sparkling look has gone out of his eyes. If he could only get somewhere by himself and lie down-provided it was not dark, he would be comfortable. He wants to be let alone; he is tired; his day's work wears him out. He comes home with a purple face, lustreless eyes, sunken countenance, tired head and mind. Any mental exertion causes fatigue. Weight in the head, distress and fullness in the head, with cold extremities. The blood mounts upward. Hemorrhages from the eyes; burning, itching and pressing in the eyes. The eyes become weak from overwork or from fine work.

Carbo veg. is one of the medicines for discharges from the ears. Offensive, watery, ichorous, acrid and excoriating discharges, especially those dating back to malaria, measles or scarlet fever, particularly to scarlet fever. A sluggish condition of the venous system. The veins seem to be most affected in all old complaints, especially whenever a patient says of himself, or a mother says of her child, that he has never been quite well since an attack of malarial fever. The daughter has never been quite well since she had the measles, or typhoid fever, or scarlet fever; Carbo veg. is one of the medicines to be thought of when symptoms are in confusion, and the patient has been so much doctored that there is no congruity left in the symptoms. Old ear discharges, or old headaches, when all the symptoms have been suppressed. It is then Carbo veg. often becomes one of the routine remedies to bring symptoms into order and to establish a more wholesome discharge from that ear. it brings about reaction, establishes a better circulation and partially cures the case, after which a better remedy may be selected.

Inflammation of the parotid glands, or mumps. When mumps change their abode, from being chilled, and go in the girl to the mammary glands, and in the boy to the testes, Carbo veg. is one of the medicines to restore order; very often it will bring the trouble back to its original place, and conduct it on through in safety.

Pains in the ear. Passive, badly-smelling discharges from the ear. Loss of hearing. Ulceration of the internal ear. Something heavy seems to lie before the ears; they seem stopped; the hearing is diminished, especially in those cases that date back to some old trouble.

The Carbo veg. patient is always suffering from coryza. He goes into a warm room, and, thinking he is going out in a minute, he keeps his overcoat on. Pretty soon he begins to get heated up, but he thinks he will go in a minute and he does not take off his coat. A procedure like that is sure to bring on a coryza. It will commence in the nose, with watery discharge, and he will sneeze, day and night. He suffers from the heat and is chilled by the cold; every draft chills him; and a warm room makes him sweat, and thus he suffers from both. He can find no comfortable place, and he goes on sneezing and blowing his nose. Perhaps he has bleeding from the nose. At night he is purplish. The coryza extends into the throat and brings on rawness and dryness in the mouth and throat. A copious watery discharge, filling the posterior nares and the throat. Then he begins to get hoarse, and in the evening he has a hoarse voice, with rawness in the larynx and throat. Rawness in the larynx on coughing; soreness to the touch. The more he coughs the worse the rawness becomes. This condition extends into the chest. Secretion of much thin mucus, finally becoming thick yellowish-green, and bad-tasting. Such is the coryza. Now, with it there comes a stomach disturbance that is commonly associated with Carbo veg. complaints. Great distension of the abdomen with gas. With this coryza he has belching, and sour, disordered stomach. Every time he disorders his stomach he is likely to get a coryza. Every time he goes into an overheated room he is likely to get a coryza, with sneezing, chest complaints, and catarrh.

This catarrhal state in the nose is only a fair example of what may occur anywhere where there is a mucous membrane. Catarrhal conditions with a flow of watery mucus and bleeding. Carbo veg. has catarrhs of the throat, nose, eyes, chest, and vagina. Old catarrhal conditions of the bladder; catarrh of the bowels and stomach. It is pre-eminently a catarrhal remedy. The woman feels best when she has more or less of a leucorrhea, it seems a sort of protection. These discharges that we meet every day are dried up and controlled by local treatments, by washes, and by local applications of every kind, and the patient put into the hands of the undertaker, or made a miserable wreck. If these catarrhal patients are not healed from within out, the discharges had better be allowed to go on. While these discharges exist the patient is comfortable. It is quite common for the Carbo veg. patient to be feverish with the coryza, but with many other complaints he is cold; cold limbs; cold face; cold body; cold skin; cold sweat. It is not so common for the earlier stages of the coryza, and the catarrhal conditions to have these cold symptoms. He is feverish in the evening and at night. But after he passes into the second stake, when the, mucus is more copious, then come the cold knees, cold nose, cold feet, and cold sweat.

The face of Carbo veg. is a great study. In the countenance and in the expression we see much that is general. The patient shows his general state in his expression, especially in the eyes. He tells you how sick he is; he tells you the threatening points. In Carbo veg. there is great pallor and coldness, with lips pinched and nose pointed and drawn in. Lips puckered, blue, livid, sickly, deathly. Face cold, pale, and covered with sweat. As the tongue is protruded for examination it is pale and cold, and the breath is cold, yet he wants to be fanned. This is true whether it be cholera, diarrhea, exhaustive sweats, or complaints after fevers. Sometimes, after a coryza has run its course and ended in the chest, there is great dyspnea, copious expectoration, exhaustive sweat, great coldness and the patient must be fanned. Cough followed by dyspnea, exhaustion, profuse sweats, with choking and rawness and he wants to be fanned. Cold face; pinched face. So the sufferings are expressed in the face. The pains and aches, and anxiety and sorrow are all expressed in the face.

The study of the face is a delightful and profitable one. The study of the faces of remedies is very profitable. It is profitable to study the faces of healthy people that you may be able to judge their intentions from their facial expressions. A man shows his business of life in his face; he shows his method of thinking, his hatreds, his longings, and his loves.

How easy it is to pick out a man who has never loved to do anything but to eat: the Epicurean face. How easy it is to pick out a man who has never loved anything but money: the miserly face. You can see the love in many of the professional faces; you can single out the student's face. These are only manifestations of the love of the life which they live. Some manifest hatred; hatred of the life in which they have been forced to live; hatred of mankind; hatred of life. In those who have been disappointed in everything they have undertaken to do we see hatred stamped upon the face. We see these things in remedies just as we see them in people. The study of the face is a most delightful one. A busy, thoughtful and observing physician has a head full of things that he can never tell: things he knows about the face. So the face expresses the remedy. In Carbo veg. the face flushes to the roots of the hair after a little wine. This is a strong characteristic. All over the body the skin will become flushed. Sometimes a flush appears in islands, which grow together and become one solid flush, creeping up into the hair. So great is the action of this remedy upon the capillary circulation that sometimes a tablespoonful of wine is sufficient to cause this flushing of the skin.

The old books talk about "scorbutic gums;" now we call it Rigg's disease: a separation of the gums from the teeth. Bleeding of the gums; sensitiveness of the gums. Separation of the gums from the teeth. The teeth get loose. We hear about "the teeth rattling in his mouth." The Carbons produce just such a state, a settling away and absorbing of the gums. They get spongy and bleed easily, and hence looseness of the teeth with bleeding of the gums, which are very sensitive. Teeth decay rapidly. Bleeding of the gums when cleaning the teeth. Teeth and gum affections from abuse of Mercury, Teeth feel too long and are sore. Drawing and tearing in the teeth. Tearing in the teeth from hot, cold or salt food; pain from both heat and cold. This is in keeping with the general venous condition of the whole system.

Sensitiveness of the tongue. Inflammation of the tongue. In certain low forms of fever, like typhus and typhoid fevers, the gums turn black; that is, they throw out a blackish, bloody, offensive, putrid exudate. If disturbed or touched they bleed; and the tongue piles up that blackish exudate - that oozing of black blood from the veins. This is present in putrid forms of fevers like the typhoid-in zymotic states. This remedy is rich in those zymotic symptoms, such as are described in common speech as "blood-poisoning." Carbo veg. is a sheet-anchor in low types of typhoid; in scarlet fever where a typhoid condition is coming upon the case, and in the last stages of collapse; in cholera, and in yellow fever at the time of collapse, where there is coldness, cold sweat, great prostration, dyspnoea - wants to be fanned. Great prostration with cold tongue.

The mouth and throat are filled with little purple aphthous ulcers, which were little white spots to begin with, but they have grown purplish and now ooze black blood. These aphthous patches bleed easily, burn and sting. Blisters form. Smarting, dryness of the mouth with bleeding aphthous ulcers. These are common features of Carbo veg. in any of the mouth and throat conditions. Tough mucus in the throat; bloody mucus in the throat. These little ulcers run together, spread and become one solid mass. A large surface will become ulcerated, denuded of its mucous membrane, and then it will bleed. Little black spots come upon it. Food cannot be swallowed because the throat is so sore. Generally the throat feels puffed.

The Cargo veg. patient has a longing for coffee, acids, sweet and salt things. Aversion to the most digestible things and the best of food. For instance, aversion to meat, and to milk which causes flatulence. Now, if I were going to manufacture a Carbo veg. constitution I would commence with his stomach. If I wanted to produce these varicose veins and the weak venous side of the heart; this fullness and congestion, and flatulence, this disordered stomach and bowels, and head and mind troubles; sluggishness of the economy. I would begin and stuff him. I would feed him with fats, with sweets, puddings, pies and sauce, and all such indigestible trash, and give him plenty of wine - then I would have the Carbo veg. patient. Do we ever have any such people to treat? Just as soon as they tell their story, you will know, enough about their lives to know that they are mince pie friends; they have lived on it for years, and now they come saying, "Oh, doctor, my stomach; just my stomach; if you will simply fix up my stomach." But what are you going to do with him? He has made himself into a Carbo veg. patient for you, and it may be quite a while before you can bring him down to a sensible diet. Now he must begin at the foot of the ladder. I only brought this up to show how a Carbo veg. patient is produced and what kind of a stomach he has, and what he has been living on. He has burning in the stomach, distension of the stomach, constant eructations, flatulence, passing offensive flatus. In reality he is in a foetid condition, a putrid condition. His sweat is offensive. He has heartburn eructations, the stomach regurgitates the food that he takes.

Carbo veg. has much vomiting at the end of the chill. Vomiting and diarrhoea. Vomiting and blood; with the vomiting of blood the body is icy cold; breath cold, The pulse is thready and intermittent. Fainting; hippocratic face; oozing of thick black blood.

Vomiting of sour, bloody, bilious masses.

There is an accumulation of flatus in the stomach, so that the stomach feels distended. All food taken into the stomach seems to turn into flatus; he is always belching and is slightly, relieved for a while by belching. Carbo veg., has cramps in the bowels and stomach; burning pain; anxiety; distension. All these symptoms are ameliorated by belching or passing flatus. Amelioration from belching seems quite a natural event; but when we study China, you will see that the patient appears to be aggravated from belching. The idea is that the patient gets relief from belching from eructation, but under Lycopodium and China it seems that no relief comes. They belch copiously and yet seem just as full of wind as ever, and sometimes even seem to be worse. The Carbo veg. patient experiences a decided relief from eructation. This is a particular symptom, but it becomes almost general, and sometimes quite general. Headaches are relieved by belching; rheumatic pains are relieved by belching; sufferings and distensions of various kinds are relieved by eructations.

This abdominal fullness aggravates all the complaints of the body. The fullness, which is described as if in the veins, is sometimes in the tissues, under the skin, so that it will crepitate. This is a feature of Carbo veg., and, in rheumatic conditions, part of the swelling is sometimes of this character. Food remains a long time in the stomach, becomes sour and putrid. It passes into the bowels and ferments further, finally passing off in the form of putrid flatus. There is colic, burning pains, distension, fullness, constricting and cramping pains from this distension. The patient complains of feeling as if the stomach were raw. This is described as a smarting, sometimes from taking food; sometimes from taking cold water. Carbo veg., has cured ulceration of the stomach. It is a deep-acting medicine, and is capable of curing all disordered conditions of the stomach; such as disorders from eating indigestible things, mince pie, too hearty food.

In Carbo veg. the liver, like all the other organs, takes on a state of torpidity and sluggishness. It becomes enlarged. The portal system is engorged, and hence hemorrhoids develop. Pain and distension in the region of the liver; sensitiveness and burning in the liver, accompanied by a bloated condition of the stomach and bowels. A feeling of tension in the region of the liver; the part feels drawn, as if too tight.

There are pressing pains in the liver, and it is sensitive to touch.

Much that I have said regarding the flatulence and fullness of the stomach applies also to the abdomen. Carbo veg. may be indicated in low forms of fever, as in septic fever, when there is a marked tympanitic condition, with diarrhoea, bloody discharges, distension and flatulence. Extremely putrid flatus escapes making the patient very offensive. A striking abdominal symptom of Carbo veg. is that the flatus collects here and there in the intestine as if it were in a lump incarcerated flatus; a constriction of the intestine will hold it in one place so that it feels like a lump or tumor, that finally disappears. Colic here and there in the abdomen from flatus. There is burning in the abdomen. No matter what the trouble is, in Carbo veg. there is always burning. The part burns; it feels full; it becomes engorged and turgid with blood. Diarrhoea, dysentery, cholera, when there is a bloody, watery stool. Cholera infantum; stool mixed with mucus; watery mucus mixed with blood. The child sinks from exhaustion, with coldness, pallor and cold sweat. The nose, face and lips are pinched and hippocratic. With all diarrheic troubles the prostration will indicate Carbo veg. as much as, if not more than, the stool. In the diarrhea of Carbo veg. all the stools, no matter what kind, are putrid, with putrid flatulence. The more thin, dark bloody mucus there is, the better is the remedy indicated. Itching, burning and rawness of the anus and round about, are strong features of Carbo veg. Soreness in all diarrheic conditions - soreness to pressure over the abdomen. Round about the anus, in children, there is excoriation. The parts are red, raw and bleeding, and they itch. Itching of the anus in adults. Ulceration of the bowels. This tendency to ulceration of mucous membranes is in keeping with the character of the remedy. Whenever there are mucous membranes there may be ulceration. Aphthous appearance. Ulceration of Peyer's glands. The patient lies in bed and oozes involuntarily a thin bloody fluid, like bloody serum.

Old chronic catarrhal conditions of the bladder, when the urine contains mucus, especially in old people, with cold face, cold extremities and cold sweat.

There is suppression of urine.

In both the male and the female organs there is a weakness and relaxation. The male organs hang down. Relaxation of the genitalia; cold and sweating genitals. The fluids escape involuntarily.

In the woman the relaxation is manifested by a dragging down sensation; dragging down of the uterus, as if the internal parts would escape. The uterus drags down so that she cannot stand on her feet. All the internal organs feel heavy and hang down.

Another strong feature of Carbo veg. is dark, oozing haemorrhage from the uterus. It is not so often a copious gushing hemorrhage, the remedy has that also - but it is an oozing. The menstrual flow will ooze from one period almost to another. The blood is putrid and dark, even black, with small clots, and considerable serum escapes with it. it says in the text: "Metrorrhagia from uterine agony." Atony is a good name for the condition; lack of tone; relaxation; weakness of the tissue. Atony is everywhere present in the Carbo veg. constitution. The muscles are tired, the limbs are tired, the whole being is tired and relaxed. This is in contradistinction to the gushing found in Belladonna, Ipecac, Secale and Hamamelis, where the blood escapes in great gushes, followed quite naturally by a contraction of the uterus, for there is more or less tonicity in connection with it. In Carbo veg., either in connection with confinement or menstruation, or in an incidental haemorrhage, the uterus does not contract. Subinvolution from mere atony; no contraction; no tonicity; weakness and relaxation. After menstruation, confinement and the various complaints that woman is subject to, there is a period of weakness that Carbo veg. often fits. When there is a retained placenta, with scanty hemorrhage - just an oozing, with no tendency to a gush of blood - the physician remembers that throughout the whole pregnancy and confinement there has been sluggishness and slowness of pains, and he says: "Why did I not think of Carbo veg. Before?" The woman has needed Carbo veg. for a month. He administers a dose, and before he has time to think about it, the uterus will expel that placenta and fix up matters so nicely that he will not need the mechanical interference that might otherwise have been necessary.

Now-a-days we hear so much about this meddlesome midwifery, this curetting, and doing this and that and the other thing, that it makes a homeopathic physician disgusted, just as if those parts were not made by Nature, and could not take care of themselves; as if they must be swabbed out and syringed out. These injections of bichlorides, etc., to keep the germs out of a woman are all nonsense. If a state of order is maintained there will be no germs. A homoeopathic physician can manage hundreds of these cases, and have no trouble. If he sees clearly beforehand what remedy the woman needs there will be no bad cases; they will all take care of themselves. Irregular contractions that bring on abnormal conditions are all avoided if the woman is turned into order before she goes into confinement. Carbo veg. is one of the medicines that prepares a woman well for confinement, that is, the symptoms calling for Carbo veg. are often present in such conditions. She is often run down, relaxed and tired. Pregnancy brings about a great many unusual conditions. There is the nausea in pregnancy; the flatulence; the offensiveness; the weakness; the enlarged veins. They will tell you that the enlargement of the veins of the lower limbs is from pressure, but it is generally not from pressure, but from weakness of the veins themselves.

Suppression of milk; prostration or great debility from nursing. It is not natural for a woman in a healthy state to become prostrated when nursing her child. She becomes so because she is sick. She was in a state of debility before she began nursing, and the weakness should be corrected by an appropriate remedy. Then she can make milk and feed her child without feeling the loss of it. Such is the state of order. Carbo veg. is a friend to the woman, and a friend to her offsprings. You will be astonished, after ten years of real homoeopathic practice, that you have so few deformed babies; that they have all grown up and prospered; that their little defects and deformities have been outgrown, and that they are more beautiful than most children, because they have been kept orderly. The doctor watches and studies him, and feeds him a little medicine now and then, that the mother suspects is sugar, to keep on the good side of the baby. She need not know that it is medicine, or that anything is the matter with the baby. So he watches the development of that little one, and grows him out of all his unhealthy tendencies. The children that grow up under the care of the homoeopathic physician will never have consumption, or Bright's disease; they are all turned into order, and they will die of old age, or be worn out properly by business cares; they will not rust out. It is the duty of the physician to watch the little ones. To save them from their inheritances and their downward tendencies is the greatest work of his life. That is worth living for. When we see these tendencies cropping out in the little ones we should never intimate - that they are due to the father or mother. It is only offensive and does no good. The physician's knowledge as to what he is doing is his own, and the greatest comfort be can get out of it is his own. He need never expect that anyone will appreciate what he has done, or what be has avoided. The physician who desires praise and sympathy for what he has done generally has no conscience. The noble, upright, truthful physician works in the night he works in the dark, he works quietly; he is not seeking for praise. He does this when called to the house, and when members of the family bring little ones to the office. In this manner children can be studied and their symptoms observed and enquired into. Whenever the mother brings the child expecting medicine, she may know that he is receiving medicine, but when she does not ask for medicine let her suspect that Johnnie is getting sugar so the doctor can get on the good side of him. That is sufficient.

In Carbo veg. the voice manifests a great many symptoms. I described a part of them when going over the coryza. I explained how it began in the nose, and traveled to the throat, the larynx, and the chest. Now many of the complaints of the larynx begin with a cold, in the nose, which finally locates permanently in the larynx and in that way we bring out the Carbo veg. cases. It is only now and then that the Carbo veg. cold settles in the larynx first; it usually travels through the nose. Most remedies have a favorite place for beginning a cold. For instance, the majority of Phosphorus colds begin in the chest or larynx. Not so with Carbo veg.; its cold generally begins in the nose, with a coryza, and the larynx is simply one of the stopping places. If the Carbo veg. cold goes down into the chest it may have its ending in the bronchial tubes or the lungs. There is a favorite place for it to settle, and it seems as if it were going to remain there. Weakness in the larynx from talking. Tired larynx of speakers and singers, and feeble, relaxed persons. The hoarseness comes on in the evening. The larynx may be fairly well in the morning, but as soon as it becomes evening his voice becomes husky. In more serious forms he may be speechless in the morning, but hoarseness and huskiness in the evening are more characteristic. Huskiness and rawness in the evening. Rawness in the larynx when coughing. Some will say there is burning, some will say rawness. Rawness in the larynx and trachea when coughing. A continual formation of mucus in the larynx, which he has to scrape and cough out. We see the same tendency to weakness in the mucous membranes. No tendency to repair; no tendency to recover. He goes on from bad to worse, with a catarrhal condition of the larynx and trachea. Hoarseness and rawness from talking, worse afternoon and evening. He is obliged to clear his throat so, many times in the evening that the larynx becomes raw and sore. Let me tell you another thing about the Materia Medica. Most of the provers were laymen, and hence there is some confusion of terms in the provings. This the physicians must see. Irritation in the throat from coughing nearly always means irritation in the larynx, though the prover said "throat." Now here is an expression, "obliged to clear his throat so often in the evening that the larynx becomes raw and sore." Clearing the throat would not make the larynx sore. Scraping the throat does not scrape the larynx; but he is obliged to clear his larynx so often that the part feels raw. Ulcerative pain, scraping and titillation in the larynx. Irritation in the larynx causing sneezing. Laryngeal phthisis. This catarrhal condition and lack of repair in the larynx goes on so long that tuberculosis begins.

Carbo veg. is one of the greatest medicines we have in the beginning of whooping cough. Its cough has all the gagging, vomiting and redness of the face found in whooping cough. It is one of our best medicines when the case is confused; when the cough indicates no remedy or when it remains in a partially developed state. A dose of Carbo veg. in such cases will improve matters very much, and minor cases of whooping cough may be wiped out in a few days. When the remedy does not cure permanently, it brings out more clearly the symptoms calling for another remedy. Most cases of whooping cough, in the care of a homoeopathic physician, will get well in a week or ten days under a carefully selected remedy. When allowed to run, they continue a long time, gradually increasing for six weeks, and then declining according to the weather. If it is in the fall, the cough will sometimes keep up all winter; so whooping cough furnishes an opportunity for the homeopathic physician to demonstrate that there is something in Homoeopathy.

The Carbo veg. patient suffers very much from difficulties of breathing. Suffocation; cannot lie down. A feeling of weakness in the chest, as if he could not get another breath. Sometimes it is due to cardiac weakness, and sometimes to stuffing up of the chest. The latter is most common. Sometimes the difficulty is asthmatic. The remedy cures asthma. We will see the patient propped up in a chair by an open window, or some members of the family may be fanning him as fast as possible. The face is cold, the nose pinched, the extremities cold and he is as pale as death. Put the hand in front of the mouth, and the breath feels cold. The breath is offensive; putrid. The extremities are cold clear to the body; not only the hands, but the whole upper extremities; and not only the feet, but the limbs clear to the body, are cold. The body only feels warm; even the skin is cold.

Carbo veg. has a rattling cough with retching and vomiting. A morning cough, with much rattling in the chest; the chest fills with mucus, and on endeavoring to expectorate he coughs and gags, or coughs and vomits. At any time during the day a peculiar choking, gagging, retching cough may develop from the mucus in the chest. He cannot get it up; it is tough, purulent, yellow and thick. Greatly reduced vitality; great relaxation; worn out persons, old people. Persons worn out from coughing or from prolonged exertion. Prostration. Catarrh of the chest, with copious expectoration.

At times there will be a hard, dry hacking cough, but finally, after prolonged coughing, it commences to loosen and he throws up great quantities of mucus. A dry, hacking cough, yet there is rattling in the chest, and the cough does not seem to do any good. He seems to cough and become exhausted, sweats and strangles. It seems as if he would suffocate with the cough. Finally he succeeds in getting up some mucus, and the follows mouthful after mouthful of thick purulent expectoration. Frequent attacks of spasmodic cough in violent paroxysm lasting for many minutes, sometimes an hour. Cold sweat, coldness and pinched appearance of the face. This increases as he goes into the paroxysm of coughing. His face looks haggard, so distressed does he become while in a paroxysm of coughing. This state is present in old phtisical cases, in the advanced stage, when they are incurable. Under such circumstances Carbo veg. furnishes an excellent palliative. It seems to strengthen the muscles of the chest so that the patient can expectorate better. It mitigates the cough; the gagging and retching and dyspnoea are relieved, and he is temporarily improved. It is a wonderful palliative in many incurable conditions with dyspnoea and weakness of the chest. In Bright's Disease, in phthisis, and in cancerous affections Carbo veg. stops the violent symptoms and mitigates greatly.

This remedy is one to begin whooping cough with. It simplifies the case greatly, and sometimes cures it in a few days. The patient coughs until the chest is sore, as if he had been beaten all over the chest. All night he has paroxysms of coughing. He sleeps into a paroxysm of, coughing, like Lachesis. He rouses up from sleep with coughing, gagging, sweating and suffocation. He will go two or three hours without a paroxysm, and then on comes one that will last an hour. He has two or three hard paroxysms of coughing during the night. He commences to fill up, he hears the rattling breathing and he knows that before long he will have a hard time of it.

This goes on and on, to the end of his life in asthmatic cases-what is called "humid asthma". Real humid asthma comes on in persons who suffer from contractions of the small bronchial tubes, so that even at the best there are little whistlings in the chest. Every time such patients take cold their whistling increases. They expectorate mucus, at first copious, then tough and finally purulent. During all this there is great asthmatic dyspnoea. Carbo veg. is an excellent remedy in all those cases of asthma where the shortness of breath is so marked that there is only a partial oxidation, as a result of which he suffers much from occipital headache and wants to be fanned. Old cases of recurrent asthma. Every time there comes a warm wet spell his asthma comes on. It is common for Carbo veg. asthma to come on in the night. He goes to, bed without warning of an oncoming attack, only. He says, "I don't like the weather;" and he wakes up with asthma. He wakes up suffocating, springs out of bed and goes to the window or wants to be fanned.

Carbo veg. is required in old, badly-treated cases of pneumonia, with a remaining bronchitis; in cases where there has been hepatization that was not cleared up, and there are bad places in the lungs and bronchial tubes, with weakness of the chest. Weakness of the chest when coughing. He feels that there is not enough force in the muscle of the chest to get up a good cough, or to help him carry on the breathing. Pneumonia, third stage, with foetid expectoration, cold breath, cold sweat, desire to be fanned. Threatened paralysis of the lungs. This is a combination of clinical states that the remedy covers well. Sometimes these asthmatic cases go on for a while, and then comes an infiltration of tubercle. If Carbo veg. can be given early it will prevent infiltration.

There is pain in the chest, and burning. Burning in the lungs; burning in the sides of the chest; burning with the cough; burning behind the sternum - the whole length of the trachea; burning aggravated when coughing; a sense of rawness even when breathing. He feels a load upon the chest, an oppression, a great weight. These are the various words that he uses, all descriptive of the same thing.

The heart comes in for a great deal of trouble. It appears to be struggling. Of course it is the venous side of the heart that is in distress. The veins are engorged. it is a venous condition of the whole patient; the veins are performing their labor with great difficulty. A state of relaxation, struggling, and there are orgasms of blood - described by some of the authors as an orgasm, by others as a tumultuous action of the heart felt throughout the body. Pulsation felt all over the body. Flushes of heat mounting upwards, ending in a sweat. Suitable, sometimes for women at the turn of life. Especially suitable to persons in advanced years.

Carbo veg. complaints come on in a weakly state in young people as if it were a premature old age in the middle-aged people; or in the breaking down that naturally belongs to old age. It is a great comforter for aged people with enlarged veins, or fullness of the veins and coldness of the extremities. Oozing of blood, with palpitation tumultuous action of the heart. The pounding goes on like a great machine, shaking the whole body.

The pulse is almost imperceptible. It seems as though the volume of blood ought to be tremendous, but it is not. Weakness of the whole vascular system. Pulse irregular, intermittent, frequent. Blood stagnates in the capillaries. Complete torper; impending paralysis of the heart. Burning in the region of the heart. With this there is an awful feeling of anxiety in the chest - in the region of the heart as if he were going to die, or as if something were going to happen. He feels that tumultuous action and tires out under it.

In going over the remedy I have said so much about the limbs, their coldness and the cold sweat, that I have practically covered most of the symptoms that belong to the extremities. Carbo veg. is an excellent remedy for the general constitutional disorder where there are indolent varicose ulcers upon the lower limbs - the legs above the ankles. There is no activity in these ulcers; thin watery discharge or it is thick, bloody and ichorous. Burning indolent ulcers; varicose, ulcers; swelling of the limbs. A gangrenous state from the extremely feeble circulation. Gangrenous condition such as old people have, senile gangrene. The limbs wither; the toes and lower parts wither and look dusky. There are blisters upon them and they ooze a bloody, watery fluid. Burning like fire. Loss of sensation. Stiffness in the joints. Excoriating sweat between the toes, and numbness. Numbness in the limb lain on. If he lies on the right side, the right hand gets numb. If he turns over on the left side, the left arm gets numb. The circulation in the part is so feeble that if there is any pressure the part becomes numb. The surface is cold. The extremities are cold. He is indolent, weak and always tired, with an aversion to mental and physical work. Every little exertion brings on a feeling as if he would faint and collapse.

The sleep is full of dreams. He wakes up with dyspnoea, wakes with cold limbs, especially cold knees. Legs drawn up during sleep. Unrefreshed after sleep. The dreams he has are the kind that most of these patients have where the remedy acts so violently upon the veins, upon the basilar portion of the brain, and upon the voluntary system. They are awful. He dreams of fire, burglars, fearful and horrible things. Anxiety, restlessness and congestion of the head prevent his going to sleep. Rush of blood to the head. His head feels hot, but to the hand the skin feels cold. The inner chest feels as if burning, but the outer chest feels cold to the hand. So it is in the abdomen. The feeling of internal heat and burning, with external coldness, is a common feature of Carbo veg.

The fever is violent; it has a violent rigor or chill. Of course during the chill he is cold, but there is one strange feature, he wants cold water during the chill, and when the fever comes on he has no thirst. That is strange; it is uncommon. It is common for patients to be thirsty when they are hot with fever, and when cold not to ask for water. It is common not to ask for water during sweat. But in this patient you observe coldness, rigor, cold breath, and even in the chill sometimes a cold sweat, and you say that it is peculiar that he drinks so much cold water. It is strange; it is uncommon; rare. Hence it is one of the strong features of Carbo veg. febrile conditions.

With the chill of this remedy one side of the body frequently feels in its natural state of heat, that is, naturally warm, while the other side, is cold. One-sided chill. Chill with icy coldness of the body. Chill with great thirst. Sweats easily, especially about the head and face Exhausting night or morning sweats. Sweat profuse, putrid or sour.

Low forms of fever like yellow fever, and a very low type of typhus and typhoid fevers. After the fever has somewhat subsided he has prolonged cold spells with lack of reaction. He does not seem to rally, but he is cold, his knees are cold, his breath is cold, cold sweat, a sort of paralytic weakness. Cadaveric aspect of the face. Cyanotic face. Coldness of the limbs. Yellow fever in the last stage, the stage of haemorrhage, with great paleness of the face. Violent headache, trembling of the body, collapse with cold breath, cold sweat, cold nose. Nose and face pinched. Vital powers very low, tells a great deal of the story of Carbo veg. Lack of reaction after some violent attack, some violent shock, some violent suffering. In weakly persons who give right out, with dyspnoea, coldness, copious sweat, exhaustion, collapse and cadaveric aspect, Carbo veg. must be given.

Carbo veg. is indicated after surgical shock, when the patient goes into collapse, and is in danger of dying from the shock of the operation. This is before inflammation sets in, for there is not vitality enough to arouse an inflammation. The heart is too weak to establish reaction enough for an inflammation. Inflammation comes after a reaction. But if reaction does not take place, Carbo veg. is one of our most important remedies.

****

Kent's comparisons of CARBO VEG arranged by
A. Gaskin in "Comparative Study on Kent's
Materia Medica"

CARBO VEGETABILIS

That is one of the first things I observed, that out side of sycotics you would seldom find a cure for asthma. There is that peculiarity that runs through sycosis which gives you a hereditary disease, and asthma corresponds to that disease. Hence it is that SIL is one of the greatest cure for asthma; it does not cure every case but when SIL corresponds to the symptoms you will be surprised how quickly it will eradicate it. While IPECAC, SPONG and ARS will correspond just as clearly to the supervening symptoms and to everything that you can find about the case, yet what will they do? They palliate; they repress the symptoms; but your asthma is no better off, your patient is not cured. ARS is one of the frequently indicated remedies for the relief of asthma; so also are BRY, IPECAC, SPONG and CARBO- VEG, but they do not cure; though they relieve surprisingly at times. Where a patient is sitting up, covered with cold sweat, wants to be fanned by somebody either side of the bed, dyspnoea is so distressing that it seems almost impossible for the patient to live longer, to another breath, then CARBO-VEG, comes in and gives immediate relief and the patient will lie down and get a very good night's rest. But what is the result? On comes the asthma again the very next cold. NAT-S goes down to bottom of this kind of case. P. 793

Think of KALI-C when after troubles like measles, a catarrhal state is left behind due to lack of reaction, the psoric sequelae. The cough following measles is very often a KALI-CARB cough. KALICARB, SULPH, CARBO-VEG, and DROSERA are perhaps more frequently indicated than other medicines in such coughs as follow pneumonia or measles. P. 635

GRAPH – From eruptions, catarrhal discharges, menstrual flow, ulcers, breath and perspiration there is marked offensiveness (like CARBO-VEG, PSORINUM, KALI PHOS, KALI ARS). P. 553

CRAVING FOR AIR IS STRONG IN THE CARBONS, yet often easily chilled and just EASILY OVERHEATED, and complaints that come on from being overheated are related to the CARBONS. P. 554

The CARBONS affect the veins more or less, relaxing and paralyzing. P. 368

PETR. is not closely related to SIL as it is to GRAPH. and CARBO-VEG, which are carbonaceous substances, and all carbonaceous products affect the back of the head. " Pain from occiput over head to forehead and eyes, with transitory blindness; he gets stiff; loses consciousness". Circumscribed pain in the occiput, aggravated on shaking the head". PETR unlike CRBO-VEG has over-sensitiveness of senses, hearing, touch and smell. P. 818

Like CARBO VEG, CARBONEUM SULPH is a most useful remedy in COLLAPSE. Marked venous stasis in organs and parts. P. 387

DIG. – constant desire to take a deep breath. When he goes to sleep the breath seems to fade away, and then he wakes up with a gasp. LACH, PHOS, CARBO VEG and some other remedies have that; remedies that affect the cerebellum particularly, producing a congestion of the cerebellum. P. 500

SPONG. – Wakens at night in great fear, and it is some time before he can rationalize his surroundings, (AESC, LYC, SAMB, LACH, PHOS, CARBO VEG). P. 983

BAR-C – A sensation of weight in the brow with headaches as if the forehead was pressing down over the eye. Like CARBO VEG, CARBO AN, and NAT MUR. P. 225

SIL – Weight in the occiput as if it would be drawn back, with rush of blood to the head, like CARBO VEG and SEPIA. P. 927

There is one class of patients you will find who will trouble you. Those cases that come into your office with puffed, venous, purple faces; they have an appearance of plethora; the face looks puffed, bloated and dropsical at times; it is a dark red, dusky face; such a face we shall cure some times with ASAFOETIDA. CARBO AN, AURUM, CARBO VEG and PULSATILLA are also related to this kind of face, but it is a very troublesome kind of face, it shows more or less cardiac disturbance and venous stasis. The venous side of heart will often be involved, when you have this kind of face. I never like to see them come into my office for they are hard cases to manage. P. 183

"Eructations relieve". "Flatulence passes upwards in quantities". Frequent eructations. Eructations do not always relieve. It is more like CHINA in its eructations. The eructations of CARBO VEG relieve for some time and he feels better. This is the way with CARBO VEG; he is distended almost to bursting and he cannot get up any wind, but finally after much pain and distention it wells up in empty eructations and then he gets relief. With CHINA he is distended and every little while getting up gas, but with no relief. It does not seem to help and sometimes patients will say they seem to get worse after it. So it is with ARG NIT at times. It evidently has both. P. 140

CHINA – Flatulent distention almost to bursting. There are constant eructations, loud and strong, and yet no relief, so extensive is the flatulence. In CARBO VEG after belching a little there is relief. LYC has both. P. 442

GRAPH – flatulence is just as marked as in CARBO VEG, and the relief from belching as just great. P. 557

KALI IOD has all the flatulence and belching of CARBO-VEG and LYC. P. 640

RUMEX – Very flatulent, full of flatulent pains; pains relieved by belching and passing flatus. (CARBO VEG). P. 887

Inflammation of parotid (mumps) changing to testes or mammae is generally cured by CARBO VEG or PULS, but ABROT has cured when these remedies have failed. P. 17

CAMPH – The air as it leaves the chest feel like that from a cellar, like CARBO VEG and VERAT. P. 256

SQILLA – has a loose morning cough and a dry evening cough (ALUM, CARBO VEG, PHOS-AC, SEP, STRAM, PULS). P. 941

Retching in an effort to expectorate is usually controlled by CARBO VEG, but SIL has it. P. 931

GRAPH – Hoarseness in the evening (like CARBO

VEG). P. 558

You remember, when we were going over the symptoms of CARBO VEG I told you that the hoarseness was worse in the evening. Now observe that the hoarseness of CAUST is worse in the morning. He gets up in the morning with a hoarse voice; if it is an ordinary case, after moving about and expectorating a little mucus, it is better. P. 304

GRAPH has cured deep-seated spinal complaints, and in such cases the patient delights to lie heavily covered in cold draft from an open window. It is easy to see in this the resemblance to CARBO VEG, which often cures when the patient wants to be fanned. P. 554

HYPERICUM – After a surgical operation, where there has been much cutting, a great state of prostration, coldness, oozing of blood, almost cold breath, of course the materia medica man, if there is one around, will say, "Why, give him CARBO VEG, of course." Yes, you will, but it will not help him. It may disappoint you. But if you are a surgeon, know your surgical therapeutics better than Materia Medica man, you will say," No, STRONTIUM CARB is what I want," it relieves that congestion all over the body; he gets warm and has comfortable night. STRONTIUM CARB is the CARBO VEG of the surgeon. P. 592

When the hay fever comes on, all the other symptoms are better, she feels nothing except the hay fever, however, all the symptoms interweave with each other. The NAT MUR symptoms will be worse in the morning and until toward noon, while in PULS they are worse in the evening, the nose filling up with the thick, yellowish-green, ropy mucus, and when the nose has been cleared a dry, burning, smarting feeling remains; if the room is warm at night she cannot sleep. NAT MUR is a little like that in the smarting and inability to sleep at night in a warm room. In NAT MUR too the discharge may continue day and night. We have an acute class in which PULS is sometimes indicated-

Copious watery discharge which ends in sneezing. In the beginning we will think of CARBO VEG, ARS, ALL-C, EUPH. With CARBO VEG there is a watery discharge and the irritation extends into the chest, with hoarseness and rawness. In ALL-C we have one group of symptoms that points to this remedy. Excoriating discharge from the nose and bland discharge from the eyes; in the larynx, sensation as if hooks were there, and sometimes this extends below the larynx; this always means ALL-C; it is also worse in warm room like PULS. The EUPH looks like ALL-C, only the discharge from the eyes is copious, watery and burning – the lachrymation burns the eyes and excoriates the cheeks; discharge from the nose is bland like PULS. Sometimes this goes into the chest, and then it is no longer EUPH. IOD is worse in a warm room; thick discharge from the nose which burns and excoriates and is yellowish-green; but there is one thing that differentiates it from all others – the patients immediately begins to emaciate when the complaints come on and he is very hungry. KALI HYDR with the thick yellowish discharge, worse in a warm room, there is a great amount of rawness and burning in the nose; external nose is very sensitive to pressure; sensitiveness in the root of the nose; whole face aches and the patient is very restless; wants to walk in open air which does not fatigue him. ARS IOD; anxiety, restlessness and weakness;

frequent sneezing and copious watery nasal discharge that burns the lip. Burning, watery discharge from the eyes like ARS. ARS wants to be very warm; wants hot water applied to the eyes; the only relief is from sniffing hot water up the nose. ARS IOD is worse in a warm room, and for days after sneezing, the discharge thickens and becomes gluey, looking like THICK, YELLOW HONEY, this excoriates; much pain through the root of the nose and eyes; often rawness in the chest with dyspnoea. The remedies having the dyspnoea are, ARSENIC, IODIDE OF ARSENIC, IODINE, KALI HYDR, and SABADILLA; these are one I have found frequently indicated in the asthmatic forms of hay fever. If the complaints have been developed after being overheated at about that time, you will find that SILICA, PULSATILLA and CARBO VEG must be carefully compared. There is another class of remedies having the stuffing up of the nose not relieved by the discharge. There is a constant desire to blow the nose, yet he gets no relief. This makes me think of LACHESIS, KALI BI, PSOR, NAJA and STICTA. PSORINUM has the copious, watery, bland discharge from the nose, it may be excoriating, and it has both. The stuffing up of the nose generally takes place in the open air; he is relieved in a warm, close room and by lying down; has some dyspnoea which is relieved by stretching the arms at right angles to the body. Hay fever is a psoric sickness. PSORINUM given in a single dose will so develop the symptoms that the case will be more clear. The attack is not the best thing to prescribe for. If it is too violent, a short acting remedy may be selected that will mitigate it. NUX VOMICA has a free, easy breathing in open air, but when he goes into a warm room his nose stuffs up, which also occurs at night, though the water drips on the pillow yet he stuffs up like PULS, BRY, and the IODINE preparations, IODIDE OF ARSENIC and CYCLAMEN. Do not understand me to have given remedies for hay fever; we cannot lay down remedies for diseases. The whole constitution must be most carefully examined. P. 863

At times a case of yellow fever gets along fairly well, but a draft causes a slight cold, and on comes sudden prostration, black vomit, death. In that case CADM SULPH competes with CARBO VEG, which used to be the main remedy in the hands of good prescribers. P. 306

Lectures on
CLINICAL MATERIA MEDICA
In Family Order

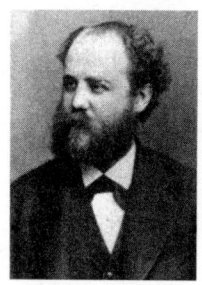

E.A. Farrington M.D.

Now I introduce to you a hidden treasure of Materia Medica. It is "Lectures on CLINICAL MATERIA MEDICA in Family Order" by Professor E.A. Farrington. I call it "hidden treasure" because it is not as largely known as Kent's or Boericke's however those practitioners who knew and studied it thoroughly, developed a deep understanding of Materia Medica. I regret for not having studied it nearly 10 early years of my practice. However now after studying it I am more confident in practice because it has covered such shortcomings in my study that bothered me for a long time. I was in this fix why we have to face failures in spite of selecting remedies on totality of symptoms or why we remain in a limited group of medicines in spite of repertorizing our cases. Failure in any case is mostly due to not arriving at the best similar remedy while missing the most suitable remedy is due to omitting some important feature or symptom of the case. Now question was what the mistake was in case taking or why important symptoms of some cases were being missed. Actually at start I studied Kent and Nash etc. who make general pictures of remedies and base the selection of medicine mainly on mental and general symptoms. But absolutely ignoring particular or pathological symptoms, because of the importance of general symptoms, is also a big mistake. I had to face a number of failures due to the same and here Farrington helped me a lot. He goes into the detail of all symptoms, into the very depth of each symptom and makes the pinpoint selection. Explanation of every important feature and symptom of a remedy with its full minuteness that we see in Farrington's Clinical Materia Medica is seldom found in any other book. It transforms a good homoeopath to a powerful prescriber and this is why Farrington is considered, like Kent, one of the great teachers of Materia Medica.

Farrington was extraordinary intelligent. Right from childhood to his college life he was respected and praised by all of students, teachers and professors because of his intelligence and love for knowledge. Dr. Korndcerfer writes in his biography,

"Having completed the prescribed course at the High School, he made a most brilliant examination and was graduated, not only at the head of his class, but with the highest average of that time attained by any graduate of the institution."

Farrington matriculated in the Homoeopathic Medical College of Pennsylvania and graduated from Hahnemann Medical College of Philadelphia in 1868. Immediately after graduation he entered practice and soon became a popular and busy physician because of his exceptional qualities and diligent nature.

He taught Materia Medica at Hahnemann Medical College where he became closer to Hering. During his teaching period he keenly worked to develop a comprehensive and easy method of studying Materia Medica. He concluded that mere reading of symptoms one by one couldn't be sufficient to understand a collective action of a medicine upon the organism. Combining and interlinking symptoms to each other could be helpful to understand the collective action of medicines and thus applying them to the similar images of diseases. One symptom of a medicine may be found in numerous other remedies but a collective picture of the action of a medicine cannot completely match to another remedy. He explains this point as,

"As we carry out the view I expressed a few minutes ago, when we examine a patient for disease, we proceed in exactly the same way as we do in case of the proving. We note the changes we see and the sensations the patient feels; we look at his tongue, we examine his urine, we put all these together and we make a pathological picture of that man. Suppose you decide the case to be one of typhoid fever. That must not be valued except by comparison, showing how the present case differs from the general disease. If the genus of the case under treatment suits the genus of Baptisia, and, if you give that remedy, the patient will recover whether you call his case typhoid fever or mumps. If this is not the case, Baptisia will do no good. If the patient has the Baptisia symptom, " thinks he is double, or all broken to pieces," that drug will not cure unless the genus of Baptisia is there too. I may be permitted to recall a remark of Carroll Dunham. At a certain consultation there was chosen for a patient, a drug which seemed to have many of his symptoms; but when Dr. Dunham was asked for his opinion as to whether that drug was the similimum, he replied, "No, I think not, for the general character of Ignatia does not correspond with the general character of the patient which does correspond to Baryta. You will find his most prominent symptoms under Baryta." One physician decided for one drug, the other for another. Each went by his study of the drug; one understood Ignatia in part, the other by its totality."

(Farrington, Clinical Materia Medica, PP. 6-7)

Farrington divides the Materia Medica into three sections being 1 Animal kingdom 2 Vegetable kingdom and 3 Mineral kingdom. These sections further have been divided into family and class order. At start of every major section as well as subdivision he describes common features of that family or class. Let us read how beautifully he describes the common features of Animal kingdom,

"Today we begin our study of the medicines obtained from the animal kingdom. I desire to preface my lecture on these remedies, with a few remarks relating to their properties in general. Many of the animal poisons are distinguished by the violence and intensity of their action, and by the decided alterations which they produce in both structure and function. The blood is often changed in its composition and quality, the nervous system suffers, and even the lower tissues are affected. The whole tendency of these remedies is to produce diseases, WHICH ARE NEVER OF A STHENIC CHARACTER, AND ALWAYS OF A DESTRUCTIVE FORM, tending thus to local as well as to general death of the body. We, therefore, look upon these poisons as medicines which suit deep-seated diseases, such, for example, as are accompanied by changes in the quality of the blood; such as profoundly affect the nervous centres. Consequently they are indicated in typhoid fevers, erysipelatous inflammations, tuberculosis of different organs and tissues of the body, and many of those dyscrasias which underlie and qualify acute diseases. You will find if you devote time to the study of this portion of the Materia Medica, more time than we can spare or than these lectures will permit, that they are often necessary to arouse vitality and direct the vital forces into a proper channel.

You will find, too, that these animal poisons are apt to affect the mind, especially the emotions. They arouse the lowest qualities in one's nature, and produce a condition which is truly shocking. Some of them arouse the filthiest lust, the most intense anger, and passions of a kindred nature. So we may find many of these drugs suitable for persons affected with insanity, whether it be the result of functional or organic cerebral changes; whether or not it be reflex from irregularities in bodily functions."

(Farrington, Clinical Materia Medica, PP. 11-12)

After giving a general view of the animal kingdom he starts his discussion on ophidian. Here again before going into details of snake remedies individually he sheds light, in general, on common action of snake poison on the organism."

"You may divide the effects of the snake-poison into three sorts: First, that which may be compared to the action of a stroke of lightning or a dose of Prussic acid. Immediately after the bite, the patient starts up with a look of anguish on his face, and then drops dead. This represents the full, unmodified, lightning rapidity of the poison. In the second form, commonly, the part bitten swells and turns, not a bright red, but rapidly to a dark purplish color, the blood becomes fluid, and the patient exhibits symptoms like those characteristic of septicaemia. The heart-beat increases in rapidity, but lessens in tone and strength. The patient becomes prostrated, and covered with a cold, clammy sweat. Dark spots appear on the body, where the blood settles into ecchymoses; the patient becomes depressed from weakness of the nervous system, or from poverty of the blood, and then sinks into a typhoid state, and dies. Or there follow nervous phenomena. The patient is seized with vertigo. Dark spots appear before the eyes; blindness; a peculiar tremor all over the body; face besotted; dyspnoea, or even stertor. Or it may assume a slower form. After the vertigo or trembling, the patient remains weak, and the place of poisoning becomes dark or gangrenous. All the discharges, the sweat, the urine and the faeces, are offensive. Dysenteric symptoms of a typhoid character show themselves. The patient goes into a low state, and finally dies. These are all phases of one action of the drug, the power of the drug to affect the blood and the nerves."

(Farrington, Clinical Materia Medica, P. 22)

After giving considerable understanding of a family/class he starts lecturing separately on remedies derived from that class. At start of a remedy he explains its general action in very

Sample Study **213**

scientific way. Let us read, for example, how beautifully he explains action of Cantharis,

"Cantharis or Spanish fly has long been used by allopaths as a counter-irritant; when applied to any part of the surface of the body, it excites a violent inflammation. This inflammation begins, of course, with erythema, rapidly advancing to vesication. The blisters thus formed are filled with a yellowish-white serum. As the inflammation progresses, they enlarge, and their contents' assume a purulent character. Finally, death of the part ensues, presuming, of course, that the application is continued long enough. At other times, large blisters termed bullae may form. These are sometimes as large as a silver half-dollar. They are raised above the surface, and are filled with a fluid which is excoriating. THIS IRRITATING PROPERTY OF CANTHARIS IS THE FOUNDATION STONE OF THE WHOLE PROVING. The pains incident to this kind of inflammation are, of course, very severe. They are of a burning character. At times when the nerves seem to be implicated in the inflammatory process, there will be sharp lancinating pains along the course of the nerve."

(Farrington, Clinical Materia Medica, PP. 85-86)

After discussing the main or general action of a remedy he notes down its comparable remedies and describes their general features along with fine differentiating details. Then he notes other important features of the remedy under discussion and again on every point he notes down the important comparative remedies describing their characteristic and differentiating symptoms. Farrington does not superficially tell the symptoms but explains the action of a medicine in quite a scientific way. He thoroughly explains physiological and pathological action and interlinks it to the characteristic symptoms of the remedy. A beautiful example of this is his description of Sepia,

"To understand the symptomatology of so large a medicine as Sepia, it having in its pathogenesis some two thousand symptoms of more or less importance, we will consider the action of the substance as it affects the various tissues. First of all the blood. Sepia causes great disturbance in the circulation; many of its symptoms seem to depend upon venous congestion, and this is especially noticeable in the portal circulation. Reviewing some of the symptoms based on this pathological condition, we find, flashes of heat which seem to begin about the trunk and go upward to the head, with anxiety, and, of course, an oppressed feeling, ending in perspiration; throbbing all over the body, particularly at the epigastrium, in the hepatic region, in the uterine region, and in the small of the back. This symptom is very common in hysteria and in chlorosis. Nosebleed, epistaxis so called, either from mechanical causes as a blow or fall, from being in a hot room, or from suppressed menses. Throbbing pain in the uterus, the uterus when examined is found to be swollen, engorged with blood, sensitive to the touch, and as we shall see when speaking of the local symptoms, displaced. The hands are hot, and the feet are cold; or, as soon as the feet become hot the hands become cold. This is an excellent indicating symptom for Sepia."

(Farrington, Clinical Materia Medica, P. 134)

Farrington, like Kent and Nash, warns, in advance, against the mistakes that can be made in the hands of most beginners. This saves the reader of many failures and develops such an accuracy in prescribing that cannot be attained by self-observation in years.

"The Majority physicians make a mistake in beginning their treatment of scarlatina. A mistake in the beginning means one of two things, either a long, tedious illness, or a short one, ending with death. The mistake is to give Belladonna in every case. Let us look for a moment at the diference between Belladonna and Lachesis..."

(Farrington, Clinical Materia Medica, PP. 66-67)

"Now, the action of Apis on the genital organs. Apis is often indicated in diseases of the female organs. Nearly all the provers experienced symptoms referable to the uterus and ovaries. It must be given cautiously during pregnancy, because if given in low potency and frequent doses it may bring about a miscarriage especially before or at the third month."

(Farrington, Clinical Materia Medica, P. 118)

In the last few years, Apocynum has come into very extensive use in the treatment of many forms of dropsy. When I give you a succinct resume of its symptoms, you will see that its indiscriminate use in dropsical conditions is by no means strictly homoeopathic. When not properly indicated symptomatically, it is necessary to exhibit it in large doses in order to produce any effect"

(Farrington, Clinical Materia Medica, PP. 179-80)

"In coughs, we sometimes find Kali carb. of use. The cough is of a paroxysmal character, and is accompanied by gagging and by vomiting of sour phlegm and of food. This suggests the use of Kali carb. in whooping cough, in which disease it has been very successful. Boenninghausen has given us a characteristic symptom for Kali carb., namely, a little sac filled with water between the upper lids and eyebrows. You will often meet with that symptom. I would warn you not to confound it with a similar condition which is in no particular pathological at all, and that is a certain looseness of the tissues in this locality occurring in persons advanced in years."

(Farrington, Clinical Materia Medica, PP. 907-8)

"Do not forget the distinction I have given you between Anacardium and Nux; I admonish you again, because I know we often give Nux when we should have given Anacardium."

(Farrington, Clinical Materia Medica, P. 249)

"I have never seen inflammation of the brain yield to Arum triphyllum, unless some one or more of these symptoms were present; either irritation about the throat, mouth, or nose, or else this peculiar picking or boring at the nose or at one spot till it bleeds. I think that it would be indicated only when the cerebral inflammation came from the suppression of some violently acting poison, such as we find present in scarlatina or diphtheria. Nor would I think of giving Arum in uraemia if it arose in the course of ordinary Bright's disease. I do not think it would be the remedy unless the symptoms already referred to are present."

(Farrington, Clinical Materia Medica, P. 237)

Along with beautiful explanations of Materia Medica Farrington denotes valuable points of philosophy that enhance our ability in correct application of Materia Medica,

"This pain in the glans penis may not be of an acute nature, but may be simply an uneasy, uncomfortable sensation. When in children, you notice this symptom, Cantharis is generally indicated; at other times, you may think also of MERCURIUS SOLUBILIS; of course, the symptom may be a habit which the child has been allowed to practice. That, of course, does not call for these remedies."

(Farrington, Clinical Materia Medica, P. 89)

"Now, let me give you the Nux vomica temperament. It does not necessarily follow that you must not use Nux if the constitution is not what I am going to describe; but it does follow that it acts better in the constitution about to be mentioned. Nux vomica suits best for rather thin, spare patients."

(Farrington, Clinical Materia Medica, P. 204)

"Another objection that has been raised against the nosodes, and one which certainly does carry some weight with it, is, that these substances do not cure, but that they interfere with the progress of homeopathy by confusing it with isopathy. So then it is said by prominent physicians within our ranks, if in a case of scrofula, you give Psorinum, your practice is not homeopathic but isopathic. I say that there is here some ground for discussion, and I hope that you will take part in the investigation of this subject. In the meanwhile, we have to fall back on the tribunal before which all prescriptions must go, and that is experience. Homeopathy is not an inductive science, in that it did not arise from a natural process of thought. Hahnemann began by experimenting. We may reason as much as we will, but we must always keep in view the facts of the case. Now, I do not know how far I would like to go into these nosodes. Correctly applied, they are not isopathic remedies. What I call pure isopathy is the practice proposed by Dr. S. Swan, of New York. For example, if a patient is so constituted that he cannot eat strawberries without being made ill thereby, he potentizes the strawberry and administers it to the patient and claims that thus the idiosyncrasy is destroyed. Isopathy rests on the bold assertion that what causes the disease will cure it when administered in a high potency. The use of the nosodes in homeopathic practice is different, because in this case we start with an experimental fact. We have taken these substances, proved them on the healthy, and have administered them at the bedside. We have found them efficacious, therefore we have the same right to claim them as medicines as we have any molecular substance."

(Farrington, Clinical Materia Medica, PP. 161-62)

"The various constitutions or dyscrasia underlying chronic and acute affections are, indeed, very numerous. As yet, we do not know them all. We do know that one of them comes in gonorrhoea, a disease which is frightfully common, so that the constitution arising from this disease is rapidly on the increase. Now I want to tell you why it is so. It is because allopathic physicians, and many homeopaths as well, do not properly cure it. I do not believe, gonorrhoea to be a local disease. If it is not properly cured, a constitutional poison which may be transmitted to the children is developed. I know, from years of experiment and observation, that gonorrhoea is a serious difficulty, and one, too, that complicates many cases that we have to treat. The same is true of syphilis in a modified degree. Gonorrhoea seems to attack the nobler tissues, the lungs, the heart, and the nervous system, all of which are reached by syphilis only after the lapse of years."

(Farrington, Clinical Materia Medica, PP. 163-64)

Such minute and fine comparison as we commonly see in Farrington's can rarely be found in any other Materia Medica. Here are some examples.

(Lachesis and Cinchona) "Bitter eructations and bitter taste belong to each; the later has the altered taste after swallowing, food retain its normal taste while being masticated."

(Farrington, Clinical Materia Medica, PP. 45-46)

"Pariera has pain going down the thighs, Berberis only in the hips and loins."

(Farrington, Clinical Materia Medica, P. 95)

Carbo veg. may cure varicose weins of the genitals, with blueness and burning-bluish tumors, Carbo animalis preferable if they are indurated."

(Farrington, Clinical Materia Medica, P. 153)

"LYCOPODIUM, which bears some resemblance to Chelidonium, is easily differentiated, especially in the rumbling of flatus in the left hypochondrium, in the sour rather than the bitter taste, in the sour vomiting, in the fulsomeness after partaking of small quantities of food, and in the character of the pains, which are dull and aching under Lycopodium, and sharp and lancinating under Chelidonium."

(Farrington, Clinical Materia Medica, P. 324)

Many times after a thorough comparative study he gives a summary of the discussion. This helps the reader retain in mind important features of the discussed remedies and easily pick out the required one when needed.

"Briefly, by way of summary:

MOSCHUS, excited, scolding, fainting; coldness; spasm of glottis and lungs.

CASTOREUM, exhausted, pains better from pressure; menstrual colic with pallor and cold sweat.

NUX MOSCHATA, errors of perception, drowsy; faints; enormous tympany; oppression of heart to throat; skin dry, cool.

VALERIANA, nerves irritated, cannot keep still; tearings, cramps, better when moving; taste of tallow or slimy.

ASAFOETIDA, reverse peristalsis, rancid eructations, offensive flatus; tightness of the chest; checked discharges.

MAGNESIA MURIATICA, faints at dinner, relief from eructations; head better from pressure and wrapping up; palpitation better on moving about; stools crumble.

MOSCHUS has been employed by allopathic physicians, when, in the course of pneumonia, a purely nervous delirium obtains. The brain is violently excited, patient talks nonsense with furious vivacity. (Trousseau.)

(Farrington, Clinical Materia Medica, PP. 129-30)

Frequently along with detailed discussions he gives shortcut clinical tips. Such tips as have a sound backup sometimes help in making very easy and successful selections,

"And we may say, in passing, only Castoreum has cured watery or green mucous stools in delicate, nervous children, who weaken under summer heat or during dentition, and who will not rally under the usual remedies."

(Farrington, Clinical Materia Medica, P. 126)

(Sepia) Clinically it has served when the servix is enlarged, with ill shaped os. Dr. Betts has had good results with it in congenital defective growth of the anterior vaginal wall, and this ill shaped os."

(Farrington, Clinical Materia Medica, P. 155)

"In addition to Nitric acid and Muriatic acid in cases having these dangerous groups of symptoms you will think of ALCOHOL. You will remember that Grauvogl found that diphtheritic membrane was dissolved and its growths destroyed by several substances, one of them being Alcohol. So this substance has become a remedy for diphtheria. Alcohol in the form of brandy and water tends not only to destroy the growth, but also aids in counteracting the terrible prostration."

(Farrington, Clinical Materia Medica, P. 238)

Farrington frequently highlights such aspects of remedies as usually are not emphasized in other books. This helps us understand maximum use of our Materia Medica and expands our therapeutic range,

"Three remedies are here to be compared with Spigelia. The first of them is MEZEREUM. This is useful in ciliary neuralgia. The pains radiate and shoot downward. There is a cold feeling in the eye as though a stream of cold air was blowing on the eye. It is especially indicated when the bones are involved, especially after the abuse of mercury."

(Farrington, Clinical Materia Medica, P. 232)

"Like Veratrum album, SABADILLA is a useful remedy on account of its mental symptoms. It may be used with success in cases of imaginary disease. For example, the patient imagines that she is pregnant when she is merely swollen from flatus ; or, that she has some horrible throat disease which will surely end fatally."

(Farrington, Clinical Materia Medica, PP. 294-95)

Another useful feature is direct and to the point use of small and rare remedies that help the reader combat such difficult and rare conditions that are not usually found in or yielded to common and polychrest remedies. Here are a few example,

"Fifth on the list is the MOMORDICA BALSAMUM, of this we have but one characteristic symptom and that is accumulation of flatus in the splenic flexure of the colon. It is a very convenient thing to know this. For instance, if during the course of a more or less chronic disease, this one symptom becomes very annoying and you do not want to destroy the action of the drug you are giving, you simply interpolate a dose of MOMORDICA, which removes the symptom and enables you to go on with the treatment as before."

(Farrington, Clinical Materia Medica, PP. 327-28)

"In cramps of the muscles you should compare Colocynth, NUX VOMICA, VERATRUM ALBUM and CHOLOS TERRAPINA. I know of no remedy better adapted to simple cramps in the muscles than the last named in the list."

(Farrington, Clinical Materia Medica, P. 332)

"ACTEA SPICATA has a special affinity for the smaller joints. It has this characteristic: The patient goes out feeling tolerably comfortable, but as he walks the joints ache and even swell."

(Farrington, Clinical Materia Medica, P. 344)

The first lecture tittled Introduction" technichally teaches us how to study and understand the Materia Medica and the therapeutic index at the end makes this wonderful book a powerful tool of homoeopathic practice.

SEPIA (I)

Belonging to the Mollusca is an animal called the SEPIA, or cuttlefish. A hard calcareous substance belonging to the cuttle-fish is, you all know, used for the feeding of birds. The animal itself possesses a little sac or pouch which contains a dark brown, almost black fluid. When pursued by larger fish, it ejects this fluid, thus clouding the water and protecting itself from its foe. This was for a long time supposed to be the only use of this fluid. It was supposed to be entirely inert when taken into the human system. Since Hahnemann's experiments have shown the fallacy of this belief, it is safe to suppose that the cuttle-fish uses it also to kill the smaller fry upon which it itself preys. The name Sepia is the common term used to designate this remedy in our materia medica, the juice just referred to being the part employed. This juice is very much used by artists. The history of the introduction of this substance into our materia medica is as follows:

Hahnemann had a friend who was an artist, who became so ill that he was scarcely able to attend to his duties. Despite Hahnemann's most careful attention, he grew no better. One day, when in his friend's studio, Hahnemann observed him using the pigment made from the Sepia, and he noticed also that the brush used was frequently moistened in the artist's mouth. Immediately, the possibility of this being the cause of the illness flashed across Hahnemann's mind. He suggested the idea to the artist, who declared positively that the Sepia paint was absolutely innocuous. At the physician's suggestion, however, the moistening of the brush in the mouth was abandoned and the artist's obscure illness shortly passed away. Hahnemann then instituted provings with the Sepiae succus. All the symptoms observed by him have since been confirmed. In 1874, the American Institute of Homeopathy, acting under the notion that our old remedies should be reproved, performed this task for Sepia. There were made some twenty-five provings of the drug in from the third to the two-hundredth potencies. These were reported at the meeting of the Association in 1875. They testify to the fact that the provings left us by Hahnemann cannot be improved upon.

Sepia is a remedy of inestimable value. It acts especially on the female organism, although it also has an action on the male. It is particularly adapted to delicate females with rather fine skin, sensitive to all impressions, usually with dark hair, although not necessarily so; the face is apt to be sallow, and the eyes surrounded by dark rings.

It acts upon the vital forces as well as upon the organic substances of the body. It very soon impresses the circulation; which becomes more and more disturbed as the proving progresses. Even as early as the fourth hour there are developed flushes of heat and ebullitions. These flushes end in sweat, with weak, faint feeling. Any motion or exertion is followed by hot spells and free sweats.

Hand in hand with this orgasm is an erethism of the nervous system, causing restlessness, anxiety, etc.

These two sets of symptoms indicate the disturbing influence of the drug upon the nervous system of animal life, and also upon the vasomotor nerves. Thence arise headaches, various local congestions, etc.

Quickly following these symptoms are those marked by relaxation of tissues and nervous weaknesses. The prover becomes languid, prostrated, faint. The joints feel weak as if they would easily become dislocated. The viscera drag, and thus originate the well-known goneness, etc. Venous congestions still continue, and, indeed, from vasomotor weakness, increase. The prolapsed uterus becomes more and more engorged, the portal stasis augments, and the liver is heavy and sluggish. The bloodvessels are full, and the limbs, hence, feel sore, bruised and tired. The general depressing influence upon the vital powers is further displayed in great weakness, faintness, trembling. Limbs feel heavy as if paralyzed; stiffness and unwieldiness of the legs, especially after sleep.

The sphincters, as well as all structures depending for power upon non-striated muscles, are weak. Hence the rectum prolapses, evacuations of bowels and bladder are tardy and sluggish, etc.; and yet there is no complete paralysis.

Organic changes are produced as exhibited in the complexion, which is yellow, earthy; in the secretions, which are offensive, sour, excoriating, etc.; in the condition of the skin, which has offensive exhalations, and is disposed to eruptions, discoloration, desquamation, ulcers, etc.

Among the conditions which modify the Sepia case, none is so important as the effect of motion. Two or three provers experienced decided relief of the symptoms (one prover excepting horseback riding) from violent exercise. But many symptoms are made worse from exertion; how, then, are we to discriminate? Since many of the symptoms arise from lax tissues, with torpidity, and, above all, with surcharged veins, exercise, by favoring the return of blood to the heart, relieves. The aggravation from horseback riding or from the motion of a ship, since it jars the sensitive parts and even tends to increase venous fulness, necessarily augments the troubles. But the headache, faint, exhausted condition, the sacro-lumbar pains, and often, too, the prolapsus uteri, are naturally intensified by walking.

Briefly, it has been found that Sepia acts well in men, or, more often, in women who are puffed or flabby, less frequently emaciated; who have a yellow, or dirty yellow-brown blotched skin; who are inclined to sweat, especially about the genitals, armpits and back, suffer with hot flashes, headaches in the morning, awaken stiff and tired, and are the subjects of diseases of the sexual organs. The man has sexual erethism, but without energy; and coitus induces great exhaustion (neurasthenia). The woman is erethistic, with hysteria, or with prolapsed uterus, palpitation, orgasm of blood, faintness, etc. In both cases, there may be portal stasis, with imperfectly acting liver, with atonic dyspepsia, sluggish bowels, uric acid deposit in the urine, and attending evidences of impaired digestion and assimilation. The general attitude is never one of strength and healthful ease, but rather of lax connective tissue, languor, and easily produced paresis.

It is to be further remembered that the Sepia symptoms are notably worse in the forenoon and evening, the afternoon bringing a time of general mitigation. Of this fact there are numerous confirmations.

We are prepared to review the symptoms in detail, and determine if they sustain the assertions thus far made.

To understand the symptomatology of so large a medicine as Sepia, it having in its pathogenesis some two thousand symptoms of more or less importance, we will consider the action of the substance as it affects the various tissues. First of all the blood. Sepia causes great disturbance in the circulation; many of its symptoms seem to depend upon venous congestion, and this is especially noticeable in the portal circulation. Reviewing some of the symptoms based on this pathological condition, we find, flashes of heat which seem to begin about the trunk and go upward to the head, with anxiety, and, of course, an oppressed feeling, ending in perspiration; throbbing all over the body, particularly at the epigastrium, in the hepatic region, in the uterine region, and in the small of the back. This symptom is very common in hysteria and in chlorosis. Nosebleed, epistaxis so called, either from mechanical causes as a blow or fall, from being in a hot room, or from suppressed menses. Throbbing pain in the uterus, the uterus when examined is found to be swollen, engorged with blood, sensitive to the touch, and as we shall see when speaking of the local symptoms, displaced. The hands are hot, and the feet are cold; or, as soon as the feet become hot the hands become cold. This is an excellent indicating symptom for Sepia.

If we look at the symptoms of the skin, again, we find its action owing to the defective venous circulation. We know that when the vaso-motor nerves are inactive, the skin is more liable to the effects of irritation, and particularly to herpetic eruptions, and it is particularly herpetic eruptions which Sepia cures. Little vesicles form, particularly about the elbow and knee joints. Ulcers may form about the joints, particularly about the joints of the, fingers. Under Sepia these are generally painless. There are only two other remedies that I know of that have this symptom, and they are BORAX and MEZEREUM. Sepia has been suggested as a remedy in herpes circinata. Sepia also causes yellow-brown spots, itching, redness, vesicles, humidity and rawness, scaling, pustules. The warm room makes the urticaria patient feel comfortable; but the warmth of the bed aggravates the pricking of the skin.

Sepia stands well in the treatment of psoriasis, though inferior to ARSENIC and ARSENICUM IODATUM.

These yellow-brown spots have also been removed by LYCOPODIUM, NUX VOMICA, and SULPHUR. CURARE is used by Dr. Baruch, of New York.

Besides Sepia, CALCAREA OSTR., BARYTA CARB., and TELLURIUM, have been recommended for ringworm. BARYTA CARB. has never been successful in my hands. TELLURIUM is useful for ringworms which seem to come in clusters.

In scabies Sepia is indicated after Sulphur, when pustules intersperse the itch vesicles.

Sepia has a marked action on the connective tissue, weakening it, and thus producing a great variety of symptoms. Thus, there is weakness of the joints, which give out readily when walking; weakness about the pit of the stomach, which is not relieved by eating and evidently the result of a sagging down of the viscera. This effect of Sepia may be utilized in cases in which the joints are readily dislocated.

Now, taking up the organs SERIATIM, we find Sepia to have a marked action on the mind. It produces a mental state which is quite characteristic, and which ought to be present when Sepia is the remedy. The patient, usually a woman, is low-spirited, sad, and cries readily. This sadness is usually associated with irritability. It will not do to find fault with the Sepia woman. At other times she manifests a condition of perfect indifference. She does not care for her household affairs or even for her own family.

This mental state of Sepia is to be distinguished from that of PULSATILLA, NATRUM MUR. and CAUSTICUM.

PULSATILLA, however, is the nearest analogue. Both it and Sepia develop a state of weeping, anxiety with ebullitions, peevish ill-humor, solicitude about health, etc. But only Pulsatilla has the mild, yielding, clinging disposition seeking consolation; but it lacks the angry irritability and the cool indifference of Sepia.

NATRUM MURIATICUM is complementary to Sepia; they agree in causing weeping mood, depression of spirits, persistent recalling of past unpleasantness, irritability, indifference, loss of memory, and alternation of mental states. The former has prominently, "worse from consolation." Clinically, we may say the same for Sepia. Both remedies, too, have ailments aggravated by vexation or anger. The two are evidently similar in causing weak and irritable nerves, but their complemental relation consists in the fact that Sepia causes the most vascular erethism; hence it is that under Sepia, disturbed feelings induce congestion to the chest and head, animated conversation causes hot face, and sweats follow excitement. In Natrum mur., the symptoms point more to nervous excitement or weakness alone, hence emotions induce tense headache, animated talking and drawing up the spine, and unpleasant thoughts cause sadness, paralytic weakness, or irritability without ebullitions. If hypochrondriacal, it is a state of melancholy from mental depression, caused by inert bowels; while in Sepia the same state depends also upon portal stasis, and therefore is more persistent and associated with more irritable temper. Natrum mur. may be called for when the mental state depends upon uterine disease or menstrual irregularity, but this will only be a prolapsus, never the uterine engorgement of Sepia. The indifference of Natrum mur. is born of hopelessness and mental languor; while that of Sepia includes an undisguised aversion to those nearest and naturally dearest.

CAUSTICUM induces sadness, especially before the menses. The face is yellow; but the anxiety is more a timid, fearful state. She is full of forebodings. She dreads the possibility of accidents to herself and others.

LILIUM TIGRINUM stands very near to Sepia. It affects the circulation, particularly the venous, and as reflex from uterine and ovarian irritation, there are, nervous irritability, must be busy, yet cannot do much; hurried manner. Depressed, full of apprehension of incurable disease, of accidents, etc. Feels that she will go crazy, weeping mood.

There is, however, an essential difference in this, that the Lilium patient finds relief in diverting her mind by busying herself; while the Sepia patient has many nervous symptoms relieved by violent exercise. It is, in the former' case, a sexual erethism which is thus relieved ; in the latter, relief is general by favoring venous circulation, nervous erethism being but slight, and being associated with lessened venereal passion.

HEPAR develops a mood which it may not be inappropriate to consider: Sadness, unpleasant events return to mind; sad evenings, even to thoughts of suicide; peevish; the slightest thing makes him break out into violence; he does not wish to see the members of his own family.

But this latter condition is not quite the indifference of Sepia. It arises more from a contrary mood. And, further, only Hepar has such violent outbursts of passion.

PLATINA is similar in its depressed moods. "Indifference; he does not seem to care whether his absent wife dies or not." But the digression is into haughtiness; or into anxiety, with fear of imminent death; or into that contracted mental state, akin to the feeling of personal superiority, in which "everything seems too narrow; with weeping mood." And, besides, as we shall see anon, the uterine symptoms differ materially.

Let us now consider the head symptoms of Sepia. There is a disease of the head called hemicrania, for which Sepia is one of our main remedies. The symptoms which indicate it here are the following: Pains over one eye (it may be either) of a throbbing character, deep, stitching pains which seem to be in the membranes of the brain, and these pains almost always shoot upwards or from within outwards. The patient can bear neither light, noise or motion. Usually, with women, there are soreness of the face and disturbance of uterine position or of menstruation. We find, too, that the patient may have a jerking of the head backwards and forwards. This has been utilized in nervous women (with hysteria for instance), and also in children with open fontanelles. In this case you should not give SULPHUR, CALCAREA, or remedies of that type. Sepia is also useful in arthritic headaches, especially when, like those of NUX VOMICA, they are worse in the morning, with nausea and vomiting. The liver is of course affected, and the urine is loaded with uric acid.

In hemicrania you may compare Sepia with BELLADONNA, SANGUINARIA, IRIS VERSICOLOR, PULSATILLA, NUX VOMICA and THERIDION.

BELLADONNA is to be selected in hemicrania when there is violent hyperaemia, with throbbing carotids, red face, intolerance of the least jar, light, or noise. It is indicated you will see in plethoric patients, and not in the cachectic as with Sepia.

SANGUINARIA produces a right-sided headache, the pains coming over from the occiput. They increase and decrease with the course of the sun, reaching their acme at mid-day. The paroxysms end with profuse urination (as in SILICEA, GELSEMIUM and VERATRUM ALBUM). They recur every seven days. Sanguinaria also has a menstrual headache which attends a profuse flow. In Sepia the menses are scanty. In Sanguinaria the pains are on the right side; in Sepia they may occur on either.

You will use IRIS VERSICOLOR in hemicrania when the attack begins with blurring of sight and the paroxysms are attended with sour, watery vomiting. The pains involve the infra-orbital and dental nerves, with stupid or stunning headache.

PULSATILLA is very similar to Sepia. Both are indicated with scanty menses, bursting, throbbing or boring, stitching pains on one side of the head, obscuration of sight, white tongue, nausea and vomiting. Pulsatilla has the most vomiting, thickly-furred tongue with clammy mouth and relief from cold air. The pains are shifting in character, and are associated with chilliness. They are worse in the evening. In Sepia, the pains recur in shocks or flashes, with proportionate increase of heat in the head; the blurring of sight is associated with heavy eyelids; and the face, though red with headache in either remedy, is ordinarily yellow with Sepia and pale with Pulsatilla.

NUX VOMICA is more suited to men than is Sepia. It cures a drawing, aching feeling as of a nail driven into the head, or as if the brain were dashed to pieces. The face is pale sallow, or sallow on a red ground. The attacks commence early in the morning, and generally increase to a frantic degree. As under Sepia, the exciting causes may be haemorrhoids, abdominal plethora, or brain fatigue. In general, however, the two drugs are very different.

ARSENICUM ALBUM will cause a throbbing, stupefying headache over the left eye. In this particular it resembles Sepia; but the prostration and restlessness of the two drugs are very different, as is also the intensity of the angry irritability, even to swearing, which Arsenicum induces. The Arsenic headache exceptionally derives a temporary relief from the application of cold water to the head.

THERIDION has, more accurately speaking, flickering before the eyes, then blurring. The nausea of this remedy is made worse by closing the eyes, and also by noise. The effect of noise is more intense than in Sepia. It seems to intensify the pains, and, as it were, penetrates to the teeth, so sensitive are the nerves to this sort of vibration.

Silicea may be needed after any unwanted exertion, if moderate. The pains excite nausea and fainting, and are followed by obscuration of vision.

Sepia is very useful in diseases of the eyes. You will find it indicated in asthenopia attending uterine diseases. You may differentiate Sepia from other remedies by the time of its aggravation, the patient generally being worse in the evening; in the morning and afternoon she is quite free from symptoms.

In conjunctivitis you will find Sepia indicated when the inflammation is of a sluggish type, occurring generally in scrofulous children. The symptoms are subacute. There is muco-purulent discharge in the morning. The eyes feel comparatively comfortable during the day, while in the evening there is an annoying dryness of the eyes.

The remaining eye-symptoms of Sepia we may summarize as follows: Cataract; trachoma; scaly lids; pustular lids with eruptions on the face; eyes irritable to light, lids close in spite of him; eyelids droop; aching, sticking pains, worse by rubbing. Causes: Uterine or liver diseases, scrofula, tea-drinking. Worse morning and evening, in hot weather, better from cold washing, and in the afternoon.

I have for years employed Sepia in blurring of sight, etc., with prolapsus uteri. (See also, Norton's OPHTHALMIA THERAPEUTICS.) I have likewise found it efficient in asthenopia, associated with exhaustion dependent upon loss of semen, whether of voluntary or of involuntary occurrence. In these respects the drug is similar to NATRUM MUR., LILIUM TIG., JABORANDI, KALI CARB. The first of these superadds muscular weakness (internal recti), stiff sensation in the muscles of the eyes on moving them, etc. There is running together of letters or stitches, but not the sudden vanishing of sight so marked in Sepia.

LILIUM TIGRINUM causes smarting of the eyes; blurring with heat in the eyelids and eyes; sharp pains over the left eye, thus symptomatically resembling Sepia. It has also burning, smarting in the eyes after reading, better in the open air, like Pulsatilla. Spasm of accommodation. (Study JABORANDI.)

CYCLAMEN and PULSATILLA may also be considered with Sepia in sudden vanishing of sight; the first with profuse and dark menses, the second with scanty dark flow. But the Cyclamen blindness accompanies a semi-lateral headache of the left temple, with pale face, nausea referred to the throat, and weak digestion.

Under PULSATILLA, which you may also use in conjunctivitis, there is a discharge, of muco-pus, but it is bland and is worse at night, with agglutination of the lids in the morning. There are fine granulations on the lids. The patient is subject to repeated highly-inflamed styes.

GRAPHITES you may employ when the canthi crack and bleed, and the edges of the lids are pale and swollen as well as scaly.

THUJA is indicated in eye affections of tea-drinkers. Brown, branlike scales accumulate about the cilia, and there are little tarsal tumors like warts.

NUX VOMICA will be called for in eye affections associated with liver diseases. The symptoms are worse in the morning, and some of them are relieved by cold bathing.

NATRUM MUR., like Sepia, is indicated in eye affections reflex from uterine disease; the lids droop. But under Natrum mur., there is more spasmodic closure of the lids in conjunctivitis, the discharges are thin and acrid; there are cracks in the canthi and also in the corners of the mouth; pains over the eyes worse when looking down.

ALUMINA likewise has falling of the lids, dryness, burning, dim sight; but Alumina has aggravation in the evening and at night. The inner canthi are affected.

Next, the action of Sepia on the abdominal organs: We find it indicated in the form of dyspepsia mentioned a few minutes ago, and also in the dyspepsia incident to uterine diseases, when it is associated with a gone, empty feeling in the epigastrium or the abdomen, with sour or bitter taste in the mouth, and with longing for acids, pickles, the gratification of the appetite for which seems to relieve these symptoms. The tongue is coated white, the bowels are usually constipated, the stools being hard, dry, and insufficient, or even if not indurated, are expelled with difficulty. The abdomen is swollen, and distended with flatus; and there is almost always soreness in the hepatic region. On making a physical exploration, you find the liver enlarged, not from fatty or amyloid degeneration, but from congestion.

Haemorrhoids are also an indication for Sepia when there is bleeding at stool, with a feeling of fulness in the rectum as though it were distended with some foreign material, which seems to excite an urging to stool. The urine has a peculiar foetid odor, and is very turbid. When standing, it deposits a lithic acid sediment, which adheres quite tenaciously to the side of the vessel.

LYCOPODIUM is a very worthy rival of Sepia in the condition just described. The distinction between the two remedies may be given you in a very few words.

A sensation of emptiness in the epigastrium is more charapteristic of Sepia; repletion after eating, of Lycopodium. Indeed, with the last-named, the repletion overshadows the other symptoms, often existing without any alterations in the appearance of the tongue. Sour taste and sour or burning eructations are, however, very common.. The abdomen is in a state of ferment. After eating, the circulation is disturbed, with irresistible drowsiness. The urine contains a sediment of free red sand. The bowels are constipated with urging and constriction of the anus. The urine, however, is not so offensive as under Sepia.

SULPHUR resembles the Sepia in many respects. Both are suited in torpid cases with defective reaction. There are abdominal plethora, congested liver, piles, constipation, hunger about 11 A.M. ; bitter or sour taste; eructations, sour or tasting like bad eggs; fulness from little food, etc. In Sulphur the face is more blotched, red, and at times spotted. Saliva nauseates him. He vomits food. He craves brandy or beer and sweets, but the latter disagree. He experiences hunger at 11 A.M.; while in Sepia it is more of a gone, faint feeling. The constipation is attended with ineffectual urging like NUX VOMICA.

For gone, empty feeling in the epigastrium, compare Sepia with CALCAREA OSTREARUM, COCCULUS, KALI CARB., STANNUM, IGNATIA, CARBO AN., SARSAPARILLA, NICCOLUM, OLEANDER, IPECAC, THEA, STAPHISAGRIA, ACTEA RAC, and HYDRASTIS.

COCCULUS has the weakness extending all over the abdomen and chest. It tires her to talk. The feeling is renewed by over-exertion and especially by loss of sleep.

KALI CARB. has empty feeling before eating, out of proportion to the feeling of vacuity caused by hunger, with undue bloating after eating, especially after soup in small quantity.

Under STANNUM, the sensation continues after eating, and extends all over the chest.

With IGNATIA, it is attended by sighing.

Under CARBO ANIMALIS, it arises from loss of vital fluids.

SARSAPARILLA has it associated with rumbling in the abdomen. NICCOLUM, without desire for food.

OLEANDER, with sensation of distended abdomen; the chest feels empty and cold.

ACTEA RACEMOSA is excellent when, with the faint, empty feeling in the epigastrium, there is a trembling, wavy sensation proceeding from the stomach over the body.

HYDRASTIS relieves when there is sinking sensation, palpitation of the heart, and mucus-coated stools.

THEA produces a gone, faint feeling; sick headache radiating from one point, and pains in the left ovary.

Gist of the Lecture

1. It acts especially on delicate female organisms.
2. Face is sallow and eyes are surrounded by dark rings.
3. There are flashes of heat and free sweats.
4. There is restlessness and anxiety.
5. Viscera drag downwards; prolapsed uterus; sensation of goneness.
6. The sphincters are weak. Rectum becomes prolapsed. Evacuations of bladder and bowels are tardy and sluggish.
7. There is relief of symptoms from violent exercise.
8. Venous congestion noticeable in the portal circulation.
9. Patients suffering from hysteria and chlorosis.
10. Throbbing pain in uterus with displacement.
11. The hands are hot and feet are cold or vice-versa.
12. Herpetic eruptions on joints.
13. Various skin ailments like yellowish-brown spots, itching, redness, vesicles, humidity and rawness, scaling, pustules.
14. Psoriasis, ringworm, scabies.
15. The patient is low-spirited, sad and cries easily.
16. Natrium mur is complementary to Sepia.
17. Hemicrania, usually left sided. Worse from motion, light, noise. Best from sleep or rest in a dark roon.
18. Very useful in asthenopia, subacute conjunctivitis and cataract.
19. Dyspepsia with empty, gone feeling.
20. Hemorrhoids with bleeding.

KEY NOTES OF LEADING REMEDIES

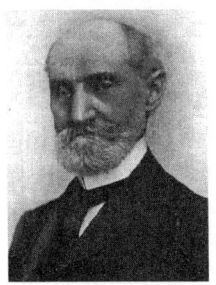

H.C. Allen

Henry Clay Allen is one of well known old homoeopaths. He was born in Canada on October 2, 1836. He graduated from Cleveland in 1861. He ran the Hering Medical College in Chicago, became president of the International Hahnemannian Association in 1886. He served as editor of the Medical Advance, taught at Homoeopathic department of the University of Michigan and at Cleveland Homoeopathic Medical College. He authored a number of well-known books as,

1. Keynotes of the Leading Remedies.
2. Keynotes with Nosodes.
3. Important Nosodes.
4. Materia Medica of Nosodes.
5. Prescriber to Allen's Keynotes.
6. Therapeutics of Intermittent Fever.
7. Therapeutics of Fevers.
8. Allen's Therapeutic notes.

Allen's Keynotes "Keynotes and Characteristics with Comparisons of Some of the Leading Remedies of Materia Medica" is considered one of the important books for beginners. As said by Gunavante,

"It furnishes important Keynotes of leading remedies and within a short compass, provides us with a number of most dependable, characteristic Keynotes and peculiar symptoms."
(Gunavante, Introduction to Homoeopathic Prescribing, P. 41)

The undimmed popularity of this book is a testimony to its practical usefulness.
(Gunavante, Introduction to Homoeopathic Prescribing, P. 246)

Allen says that the life work of the student of the Homoeopathic Materia Medica is one of constant comparison and differentiation. He must compare the pathogenesis of a remedy with the recorded anamnesis of the patient; he must differentiate the apparently similar symptoms of two or more medicinal agents in order to select the similimum. For this purpose, he says, the student or the practitioner must have knowledge of the individuality of the remedy; something that is peculiar, uncommon, or sufficiently characteristic that may be used as a pivotal point of comparison.

(Allen, Keynotes, P. 5)

So he hopes his work "Keynotes" will benefit the beginners in this sphere and it really does.

He describes his purpose of presenting this book to the profession as under,

"An attempt to render the student's task less difficult, to simplify his study, to make it both interesting and useful, to place its mastery within the reach of every intelligent man or woman in the profession, is the apology for the addition of another monograph to our present work of reference."

(Allen, Keynotes, P. 6)

Here we should understand an important point that the true purpose of "Keynotes" as pointed out by Allen himself, is to use them for comparison in order to find the most similar remedy; not to base the selection solely on one or two of them. Unfortunately many people in homoeopathic circles misuse

"Keynotes" as pointed out in the chapter "Symptoms". They try to select the remedy on one or a few of Keynote symptoms that mostly results in failures. If a lady comes to us with complaints of scanty menses, dysmenorrhoea and rheumatic pains agg. by lying and amel. by motion, we may think of Pulsatilla. But numerous other remedies have these symptoms. So if she is inclined to weeping, is mild yielding, warm blooded and usually thirstless, then she is Pulsatilla. If she has dread of bathing and coition, ravenous hunger and is amel. by physical exertion; she would be cured by Sepia. Further, if she is inclined to obesity, is always sad, has a chronic constipation and cannot bear either heat or cold then she would be Graphites. This is correct use of keynote symptoms. That is, if a remedy seems to be indicated by a few symptoms we may confirm it by its keynotes because they are its fundamental and pivotal symptoms. Reversely if we base the selection on some keynotes, instead of the totality of the symptoms it would mostly result in failure. Remember, selection always must be on the totality--- the whole case. Let us read a remedy from Allen's "Keynotes".

PULSATILLA

Anemone   *Ranunculaceae*

Adapted to persons of indecisive, slow, phelgmatic temperament; sandy hair, blue eyes, pale face, easily moved to laughter or tears; affectionate, mild, gentle, timid, yielding disposition - the woman's remedy.

Weeps easily: almost impossible to detail her ailments without weeping (weeps when thanked, Lyc.).

Especially, in diseases of women and children.

Women inclined to be fleshy, with scanty and protracted menstruation (Graph.).

The first serious impairment of health is referred to puberic age, have "never been well since" - anaemia, chlorosis, bronchitis, phthisis.

Secretions from all mucus membranes are thick, bland and yellowish- green (Kali s., Nat. s.).

Symptoms ever changing: no two chills, no two stools, no two attacks alike; very well one hour, very miserable the next; apparently contradictory (Ign.).

Pains: drawing, tearing, erratic, **rapidly shifting** from one part to another (Kali bi., Lac c., Mang. a.); are accompanied with constant chilliness; the more severe the pain, the more severe the chill; appear suddenly, leave gradually, or tension much increases until very acute and then "lets up with a snap;" on first motion (Rhus).

Thirstlessness with nearly all complaints; gastric difficulties from eating rich food, cake, pastry, especially after pork or sausage; the sight or even the thought of pork causes disgust; "bad taste" in the morning.

Great dryness of mouth in the morning, without thirst (Nux m. - mouth moist, intense thirst, Mer.).

Mumps; metastasis to mammae or testicle.

"All-gone" sensation in stomach, in tea drinkers especially.

Diarrhoea: only, or usually at night, watery, greenish-yellow, very changeable; soon as they eat; from fruit, cold food or drinks, ice-cream (Ars., Bry.; eating pears, Ver., China; onions, Thuja; oysters, Brom., Lyc.; milk, Cal., Nat. c., Nic., Sul.; drinking impure water, Camp., Zing.).

Derangements at puberty; menses, suppressed from getting feet wet; too late, scanty, slimy, painful, irregular, intermitting flow, with evening chilliness; with intense pain and great restlessness and tossing about (Mag. p.); flows more during day (on lying down, Kreos.). Delayed first menstruation.

Sleep: wide awake in the evening, does not want to go to bed; first sleep restless, sound asleep when it is time to getup; wakes languid, unrefreshed (rev. of, Nux).

Styes: especially on upper lid; from eating fat, greasy, rich food or pork (compare, Lyc., Sulph.).

Threatened abortion; flow ceases and then returns with increased force; pains spasmodic, excite suffocation and fainting; must have fresh air.

Toothache: relieved by holding cold water in the mouth (Bry, Coff.); worse from warm things and heat of room.

Unable to breathe well, or is chilly in a warm room.

Nervousness, intensely felt about the ankles.

Relations. - Complementary: Kali m., Lyc., Sil., Sulph. ac.; Kali m. is its chemical analogue.

Silicea is the chronic of Pulsatilla in nearly all ailments. Follows, and is followed by, Kali m.

One of the best remedies with which to begin the treatment of a chronic case (Cal., Sulph.).

Patients, anaemic or chlorotic, who have taken much iron, quinine and tonics, even years before.

Ailments: from abuse of chamomile, quinine, mercury, tea-drinking, Sulphur.

Follows well: after, Kali bi, Lyc, Sep, Sil, Sulph.

Aggravation. - In a warm close room; evening, at twilight; on beginning to move; lying on the left, or on the painless side; very rich, fat, indigestible food; pressure on the well side if it be made toward the diseased side; warm applications; heat (Kali m.).

Amelioration. - In the open air; lying on painful side (Bry.); cold air or cool room; eating or drinking cold things; cold applications (Kali m.)

KEYNOTES OF THE HOMOEOPATHIC MATERIA MEDICA

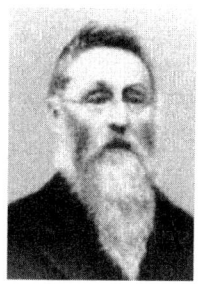

Dr. Adolph Von Lippe

Lippe, a Hahnemann's pupil, is one of great men of Homoeopathic Materia Medica. His full name was Adolphus Graf zur Lippe-Weissenfeild. He was born on 5 November 1812 in Germany. He was the eldest son of the late Count Ludwid and Countess Augusta zur Lippe and was destined by them for the profession of law. He, therefore, finished his academic preparations and graduated from the University of Berlin. But during his legal studies he was attracted to Homoeopathy and afterwards he devoted himself to it.

He was one of the first graduates of Allentown. With Hering and Raue he taught at Hahnemann Medical College, Philadelphia. He was one of the founders of the International Hahnemannian Association. He was one of the finest homoeopaths. Constantine Lippe was his son.

His major literary work was Lippe's Materia Medica. Dr. Von Lippe filled the chair of materia medica in the Homoeopathic College of Pennsylvania from 1863 to 1868 and with distinguished success. He also translated valuable Italian, German, and French Homoeopathic essays and treatises that are now standard. He died on 28 January 1888.

Gunavante, in his "Introduction to Homoeopathic Prescribing" introduces Lippe's "Keynotes and Redline Symptoms" as follows,

"Lippe is held in high esteem as a prescriber of unique ability wherever homoeopathy is practiced. This book contains not only the key-notes which Dr. Lippe found useful; but the key-notes brought to the notice of the profession by many other authors as well. As such, it is very useful book of reference and study"

(Gunavante, Introduction to Homoeopathic Prescribing, P. 253)

This classical handy book contains 350 remedies including all poluchrests and some rares. Three types of letters, blocks, italics and romans, have been used to indicate relative value of symptoms. While describing a symptom Lippe very masterly introduces comparable remedies in brackets. He also mentions the names (abbreviations) of provers after every symptom which highlight authenticity of the book.

NATRUM MURIATICUM

COMMON NAMES: Common Salt : Chloride of Sodium

Often of great benefit in the treatment of malarial disease and intermittent fevers.

Hard chill about 11 A.M., with great thirst which continues through all stages ; the heat is characterized by the most violent headache [Ra].

Continued chilliness and want of animal heat very marked (Nux-v., Sil.).

Intermittent fever, made inveterate by the use of quinine (Apis, Ars., Ign., Ipec., Nux-v., Puls., Sep., Sulph.) [N.].

Pulse intermitting (Dig., Ign.).

Twitching in the muscles and limbs (Bell., Cupr., Kali-p., Mag-p., Stram.).

Shortening of muscles (Amm-m., Caust., Sil.).

Painful contraction of the hamstrings [He.].

Great coldness of the body, with disposition to put on more clothing.

INTERMITTENT FEVER, WITH SPLITTING HEADACHE (Nux-v.).

The most weakness is felt in the morning, in bed (Ambr., Carb-v., Con., Puls.).

Continuous heat in the afternoon, with violent headache and unconsciousness.

Intermittent fever, from living in damp regions [D.].

Great weakness and debility of mind and body after exertion.

Every movement accelerates the circulation (Bry., Dig.,).

GREAT EMACIATION (Abrot., Calc-p., Op., Sars., Sanic., Sil.,).

Great emaciation while living well ; especially seen in the neck [N.].

CHILL AT 10 TO 11 A.M. (Agagr., Ars., Carb-v., Lob., Nux-v., Sulph. [N.].

Continuous chilliness from morning till noon.

Any fever with violent headache, heat in the face and great thirst. If it is regularly aggravated at 10 to 11 A.M. [N.].

There is vomiting with the chill (Eup-p) [D.].

Complete relief during sweat (Ars.). [N.].

Sallow complexion or very pale countenance [Bt.].

After great bodily exertion an itching nettle-rash appears [N.].

Hang-nails : skin around the nail dry and cracked [N.].

Congestion of blood to the head, chest and stomach, with coldness of the legs (Bell., Stram.).

SPLITTING HEADACHE (Bry., Glon.).

Hammering in the front region on the head [D.].

Headache accompanied by constipation (Bry.,) [D.].

Headache as if bursting ; beating or sticking through to the neck and chest, with heat in the head, red face, nausea and vomiting before, during or after catamania, or during the fever stage, decreasing gradually after the sweat [N.].

School-girls' headache (Calc-p) [N.].

Useful (in eye diseases) after all kinds of cauterization with Arg-n. [N.].

Unsteadiness of vision ; objects become confused, on looking at them ; letters and stitches run together [N.].

Drawing, stiff sensation in the muscles of eyes, on moving them [N.].

Of value in bringing up power of vision, after debilitating illness (Chin.).

Excessively sore, red disgusting eye-lids [Ra.].

Asthenopia (Calc-p., Phos., Rut., Sep.).

CILIARY NEURALGIA, WHICH COMES ANS GOES WITH THE SUN (Spig.) [D.].

Blepharitis (Bor., Euphr., Graph., Sulph.). [D.].

Lachrymation and scalding tears [D.].

Bad effect from anger (Bry., Ign., Nux-v., Staph.) and illness induced from talking.

Dryness of the vagina, which is painful during an embrace (Graph., L yc., Sep.) [G.].

Very sad and gloomy during the menses, with much palpitation of the heart and morning headache [G.].

SCANTY AND DELAYED MESTRUATION--- IS A PROMINENT INDICATION FOR THE USE OF THIS SALT [Bt.].

WATERY LEUCORRHOEA (Graph., Nit-ac., Puls.) [D.].

Especially useful in uterine toubles, accompanied by backache, which relived by lying on the back, or on something hard [D.].

Every morning pressing and pushing towards the genitals ; has to sit to prevent prolapse (Sep.) [N.].

Cutting in the urethra, after micturation (Berb., Calc-p., Canth., Con., Dig., Lyc., Petros., Rhus-T., Sulph.) [N.].

Catarrh of bladder, with burning on urinating (Hydr., Kali-B., Lyc.) [D.].

Pain in the urethra, just after urinating (Sars.).

Has to wait a long time for the urine to pass, if others are present [Br.].

SEMINAL EMISSION EVEN AFTER COITUS [Br.].

Gleet : clear mucus ; chronic, after absue of Arn-Nit.(or Nitrate of Silver) [N.].

Averse to coition, or painful coition [B.].

Hair falling of pubes [N.].

PAIN IN THE BACK, AS IF BROKEN, RELIEVED BY LYING ON SOMETHING [N.].

Chlorosis : chronic cases ; cachetic individuals, with dead, dirty skin ; frequent palpitation and fluttering of the heart ; oppression and anxiety in the chest [G.].

Herpetic eruptions of little, watery blisters (Rhus-T.) [D.].

Eruptions on the flexor surfaces (eruptions on the extensor surfaces—Kreos.) [D.].

Warts on the palms of hands [N.].

Itching eruptions, dry or moist ; worse at the roots of the hairs (Rhus-T.) [N.].

Tormenting sleeplessness, after gnawing grief (Ign., Kali-Br.) [N.].

Frequent dreams of robbers in the house, and on waking will not believe the contrary, until a search is made [N.].

AGGRAVATION: In the morning; at night; from 10 to 11 A.M. ; on lying down, especially on the left side ; from heat in general ; from the heat of sun ; after abuse of quinine ; during hot weather ; at sea-shore ; from mental exertion ; and from noises.

AMELIORATION: By sweat ; in the open air ; from cold bathing ; from lying on right side ; from pressure ; from tight clothing ; and while fasting.

RELATIONSHIP

COMPARE: Alum., Apis., Ars., Bry., Calc., Carb-V., Chin., Dig., Euphr., Ferr., Graph., Hydr., Ign., Ipec., Kali-P., Lach., Lyc., Merc., Mur-Ac., Nit-Ac., Nux-V., Op., Petr., Phos., Plb., Puls., Rhus-T., Sep., Sil., Sulph., Thuj., Urt., Vetr. and Zinc.

COMPLEMENTARY TO: Apis., Ign. and Sep.

ANTIDOTES: Ars., Phos., and Nit-Sp-D.

ANTIDOTES: Apis., Arg-N., and Quin.

DOSAGE : 30 to 200 and higher potencies. In frequent doses higher potencies give better results.

THE GENIUS OF HOMOEOPATHIC REMEDIES

****

By S.M. Gunavante

S.M. Gunavante was one of very laborious and zealous Indian Homoeopaths. He was born in North Karana (India) in 1915, had his schooling in Honava. He was a brilliant student and used to top the class in his school. He could not pursue his studies due to pecuniary difficulties and took up a job in an insurance company.

During his professional career his friend Dr. G.L Koppikar generated his interest in Homoeopathy. He studied Homoeopathy deeply after his retirement. At this stage he came in touch with Dr. Bhanu D. Desai and assisted him in compiling his books like "How to Find the Similimum With Boger-Boeninghausen's Repertory" and "Bring up Healthy Children with Homoeopathy". Dr. Gunavante has contributed following books and treatises to the literature of Homoeopathy.

1. Introduction to Homoeopathic Prescribing.
2. Probing the Mind and Other Guiding Symptoms.
3. Perceiving Crucial Symptoms.
4. The Genius of Homoeopathic Remedies.
5. Amazing Power of Homoeopathy.
6. How to be a Good Homoeopathic Healer.

As said before, one should start studying the Homoeopathic Materia Medica from such books which provide basic, essential and precise knowledge in an easy and brief way. S.M. Gunavante in "The Genius of Homoeopathic Remedies" has successfully met this need of beginners.

This book covers 101 remedies including the most commonly used and some rares like Latrodectus Mactans and Vipra. Important features of the included remedies, called by the author "Minimum Syndrome of the Maximum Value", have been furnished in a comprehensive and concise manner. A remedy divided into 11-12 sections, each of them important clear and concise, becomes easily retainable for the beginner. He describes, in the Preface, how he arranges symptoms of a remedy in this beautiful book,

"It is thus that I went on collecting the most peculiar symptoms of remedies. In the beginning this effort was limited to what is described hereafter as the "Synopsis" and the "Mind". Very soon I found that the "Causation", "Modalities" and "Cravings and Aversions" are equally indispensable. The sections on "Female/male" complaints as well as those of the "Child" were then felt to be necessary. The last section on "Peculiar, Uncommon" symptoms (relating primarily to "Particulars" was added, initially with reluctance (as they are "mere" particulars), but which on deeper reflection were felt to be as indispensable as others provided they are Peculiar and Uncommon. The section III "Objective Symptoms" was added last as they too are capable of putting us on the track of the simillimum.

It was also felt that the only way to make the readers study and master the "Genius" of each remedy was to give cases and challenge them to find the solution. Hence the addition of "Case Studies".

(Gunavante, The Genius of Homoeopathic Remedies, PP. V, VI)

SULPHUR

Keywords: An unclean, lazy, egotistical philosopher with burnings of hell-fire all over.

1. Synopsis (Identifying Features)

1. Indifference to personal appearance – dirty, filthy, puts on "threadbare clothes and battered hats".
2. Those who are lean, stooped-shouldered and walk and sit stooped. Drop into a chair because standing is the worst position.
3. Cannot stand hunger; famished before meals; especially at 11a.m. must have something to eat.
4. Averse to heat – intolerant of much clothing throws off bedclothes.
5. Craving for fats, sweets, alcoholic drinks.
6. Speculates on religious or philosophical subject; "ragged philosopher". Indifference about the lot of others. Selfish.
7. Egotist – foolish happiness and pride. Thinks himself to be in possession of beautiful things; everything looks pretty which the person takes a fancy to.
8. They are not disturbed by uncleanliness; yet are oversensitive to filthy odours. Have a desire to wash.
9. Burning sensation in various parts (one of Nash's burning trio). Constant heat on top of head, while the feet are cold. Burning of palms, soles. Burning in urethra after coition or when semen is discharged. Burning in bowels, in rectum, in eruptions after scratching. Flushes of heat at climacteric.
10. Redness: Orifices of the body are very red; red anus, red mouth of urethra; lips bright red as if blood would burst through. Red eyelids, ear or nostrils.
11. Itching violent, voluptuous (feels pleasant when scratching); but burning follows scratching. Sensitive to washing.

12. Puts feet out of bed at night to keep them cool.
13. Drinks much, eats little. Has to get up at night to eat.
14. Sleeps in catnaps; irresistible sleepiness during the day; wakeful whole night. Disturbed (wakens) at the slightest noise.
15. Skin: Apt to be hard, rough, coarse and measly; offensive smell despite frequent washing.

2. Mind

Unclean body and habits. Quick tempered, quick motioned. Quarrelsome. Egotism. Peevish, mean and selfish; no regard for others. Slow, lazy, and hungry; always tired; averse to work. Highly emotional, religious, philosophical dreamer. Delusion he is wealthy. Timidity. Capricious, discontented. Indolent, averse to work. Prostration of mind. Suspicious; taciturn. Causeless weeping.

3. Objective

Redness of orifices or single parts. Stooped-shouldered; cannot walk erect. Face dirty looking; hair uncut; indifference to dress. Emaciation. Soreness in folds of skin. Local burning or congestions—soles, vertex; sticks feet out of bed at night. Cannot stand hunger for long – sudden hunger and weakness, esp. at 11a.m. Skin unhealthy, festers; does not heal. Impatient; egotistic.

4. Causation (A.F.)

Suppression of skin eruptions. History of excessive sexual indulgence; masturbation, suppression of discharges; ill effects of vaccination.

5. Modalities

Agg: Suppression; bathing and washing; weather changes. Periodicity: 11a.m., weekly, full moon. Standing; during climax. Warmth of bed; early morning; night.

Amel: Dry, warm weather. Lying on right side. Open air.

6. Food & Drinks

Appetite, Thirst

Appetite lost, or excessive. Eats little and drinks much. Great acidity, sour eructations; burning in stomach. Suddenly hungry and faint at 11 a.m., must eat.

Desire: Great for sweets, alcoholic drinks; apples; cold drinks; milk.

Disagrees: Milk, sweets, raw food; sour apples.

Aversion; Bread; fat and rich food; tobacco; meat.

7. Female

Menses acrid make parts burn. Vagina burns. Burning leucorrhoea too, and excoriating; nipples crack, smart and burn. Sterility with too early, copious menses. Never been well since that miscarriage. Puerperal septicaemia; after suppressed lochia (Pyro). Phlegmasia alba dolens – Pruritus pudenda. Movement in abdomen as if a child. Pseudo pregnancy (Croc., Thu.).

Male: Sexual weakness from orgasm. Penis cold, relaxed, powerless; semen thin watery inodorous.

8. Child

Lips bright red, complexion sallow. Restless, hot and kicks off the clothes at night. Emaciated with old looking face, big belly, dry, flabby skin. Child grasps everything with in reach and thrusts it into its mouth. Stool is large and painful. Child is afraid to have a stool on account of pain; it desists on first effort. Fontanels close too late. Child dreads to be washed or bathed (in cold water : Ant-c.).

9. Peculiar Uncommon, Grand Characteristics

1. Mouth - Tongue dry, red at the edges and tip.
2. Rectum - Diarrhoea after midnight, painless; driving out of bed in the morning(Aloe., Psor.).
3. Rectum - Itching, burning; haemorrhoids wit burning and sticking; congestion.
4. Stool - Both discharge of urine and discharge of faeces are painful to parts over they pass.
5. Stool - Discharge of prostatic fluid after passing urine and stool.
6. Gen. Female - When complaints relapse continually (menses, leucorrhoea, etc.), patient seems to get well when the disease returns again and again.
7. Chest - Haemorrhoids suppressed - with colic, palpitation, congestion to lungs; back feels stiff as if bruised.
8. Chest - Sharp pain at heart going through chest to between shoulders, esp. with dyspeptic symptoms.
9. Back - Pain in small of back; was obliged to walk bent over; violent pain on stooping, on rising from a seat.
10. Sleep - Wakes up singing due to happy dreams on the previous day.
11. Dreams - Of wild animals; clairvoyant; danger; disease; falling from high places; fire; ghosts; specters; murder; misfortune; wild beasts; vexation.

12. Sleep -	Dreams; vivid; anxious, horrible, with great palpitation; that he has been bitten by dog; that he is falling.
13. Skin -	Dry, offensive, easily bleeding, burning eruptions; begin on back of head and behind ears; pains and cracks; amel. by scratching. Also eruptions humid, offensive with thick pus, yellow crusts, bleeding and burning.
14. General -	Alternation of complaints; pale and red cheeks; diarrhoea and constipation; asthma or gout and skin eruptions.
15. General -	Facilitates absorption of serous or inflamatory exudates in brain, pleura, lungs, joints, when Bry., Kali mur or well selected remedy fails.
16. General -	Hot flushes at climacteric period, with hot head, hands and feet, and a great gone-ness in stomach.
17. General -	Lack of reaction. When carefully selected remedies fail Sulph. will arouse the reactive energy of the system; will prepare the way for some other remedy; esp. in acute cases(chronic:Psor.).

CASES

Sulphur

Lachrymation in the morning (KR.245); Photophobia (K.R.261); Eyes red (K.R 264); Vision dim (KR 275); Opacity of cornea (KR. 247); Menses late (KR. 727); and scanty (KR. 728).

POCKET MANUAL OF THE HOMOEOPATHIC MATERIA MEDICA

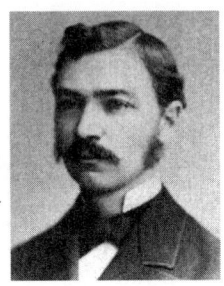

William Boericke, M.D.

Homoeopathic profession owes great debt to Dr. William Boericke for preserving and translating into English the sixth edition of the Organon--- the ripe fruit of the life work of our venerable master.

Boericke was born in Austria in 1849 and received his primary education in the public schools of Cincinnati, Ohio. He graduated in 1863 and then engaged in the Homoeopathic pharmaceutics with the celebrated firm Boericke & Tafel in Philadelphia. In 1876 he entered the Hahnemann Medical College where he was graduated in 1880. He served as editor of the California Homoeopath, founded the Pacific Coast Journal of Homoeopathy and edited it until 1915. He was one of incorporators of the Hahnemann College. He was a member of the California State Homoeopathic Society, and of the American Institute of Homoeopathy. Dr. Boericke was one of the board of trustees of Hahnemann College Hospital. Besides translation of Organon's sixth edition William Boericke presented the following books to the profession.

1. Pocket Manual of Materia Medica with Repertory.
2. A Compend of the Principles of Homoeopathy.
3. Regionals of the Boericke's Materia Medica.

Boericke's Pocket Manual of Materia Medica became so popular that it went through 9 editions in life of the author. Basically it is a reference book but when the reader is well acquainted with the principles of Homoeopathy and values of different types of symptoms, it is equally a useful study book of Materia Medica. The book covers over 600 remedies including all polychrests and many rares. Two types of letters, roman and italic, have been used to indicate relative value of symptoms. He starts a remedy by describing its general action followed by its symptoms in schematic form. While describing symptoms he mentions comparable remedies so that the reader compare relevant remedies. It is a comprehensive and handy book for day to day practice; used by beginning and experienced homoeopaths. It also contains a useful reportorial section as well as a therapeutic index. Essential information of the included remedies has been given in a compact form. Boericke says,

"In its present compact form it contains the maximum number of reliable Materia Medica facts in the minimum space."

(Boericke, Pocket Manual of Materia Medica, Preface)

Regarding Boericke's Materia Medica beginners must know that it contains some medicines not fully proved according to homoeopathic principles. Such remedies are devoid of characteristic and individualizing symptoms upon which a homoeopathic selection always depends. We know that proving on healthy human beings is one of the basic principles of homoeopathy. We must abide by the principles. They are universal laws and we cannot practice homoeopathy confidently and successfully without following the laws. Characteristic and individualizing symptoms cannot be achieved/known without thorough provings and a confident and successful prescription cannot be secured without such symptoms. Thus, being homoeopaths, we can rely only on those remedies which have been well proved and their characteristic and individualizing symptoms have been known. Those remedies which have only pathological or common symptoms are useless for homoeopathic purposes. Many people in homoeopathic circles use unproved medicines. I feel pity for those ignorant fellows who take non-homoeopathic medicines for homoeopathic ones and blame homoeopathy for the consequent failures. This happens due to lack of knowledge. When we have knowledge of well proved medicines and prescribe them precisely according to the law of similia similibus curentur the success is sure. We must have a sound and confident basis for prescription to be confident of cure.

On the other hand if we prescribe only on pathological symptoms (without characteristic and individualizing ones) based on the so-called pathological reports of the Materia Medica, then failures will be unavoidable. Many people prescribe such medicines as Passiflora for insomnia, Avena Sativa for nervous weakness, Echinacea for septic conditions and so on. Each of such pathological and common things is due to numerous causes and accompanied with varied symptoms. How a medicine can cure a disease in different patients with different causes and symptoms. Medicines devoid of characteristic and differentiating symptoms cannot be used for homoeopathic purposes and unproved medicines are not homoeopathic at all. Boericke has not introduced or suggested such medicines for homoeopathic practice. He has mentioned them only for the sake of future provings. If a remedy happens to produce clear, characteristic and homoeopathically essential symptoms then it can be used for homoeopathic purposes. But this is neither practicable nor advisable for beginners. This can be done with extensive knowledge and lot of experience. Thus beginners are strongly advised to follow the law and bring into practice only well proved remedies so that they may be sure of results. Boericke makes his plea for including unproved medicines into his Materia Medica as follows,

"I have tried to give a succinct resume of the symptomatology of every medicine used in Homoeopathy, including also clinical suggestions of many drugs so far not yet based on provings, thus offering the opportunity to experiment with these and by future provings discover their distinctive use and so enlarging our armamentarium.

I am aware that there is a difference of opinion about the advisability of further introduction of remedies, especially of such as seem obsolete or to some minds illusory. But it is not for the compiler to leave out any substance that received the clinical endorsement from a reliable source."

(Boericke, Pocket Manual of Materia Medica, Preface)

Now we have a more developed and practical book of Boericke's style. It is Frans Vermeulen's "Concordant Materia Materia Medica". Vermuelen has collected symptoms from Boericke, Boger, Clarke, Lippe, Phatak, Pulford, Cowperthwaite, Allen and Kent and compiled them in such a way that all the authentic material of these books has become available to the reader without repetition. So Vermeulen's Materia Medica being categorically like that of Boericke has become a more practical book.

LYCOPODIUM CLAVATUM (CLUB MOSS)

This drug is inert until the spores are crushed. Its wonderful medicinal properties are only disclosed by trituration and succussion.

In nearly all cases where Lycopodium is the remedy, some evidence of urinary or digestive disturbance will be found. Corresponds to Grauvogle's carbo-nitrogenoid constitution, the non-eliminative lithaemic. Lycopodium is adapted more especially to ailments gradually developing, functional power weakening, with failures of the digestive powers, where the function of the liver is seriously disturbed.

Atony. Malnutrition. Mild temperaments of lymphatic constitution, with catarrhal tendencies; older persons, where the skin shows yellowish spots, earthy complexion, uric acid diathesis, etc; also precocious, weakly children. Symptoms characteristically run from right to left, acts especially on right side of body, and are worse from about 4 to 8 pm. In kidney affections, red sand in urine, backache, in renal region; worse before urination. Intolerant of cold drinks; craves everything warm. Best adapted to persons intellectually keen, but of weak, muscular power. Deep-seated, progressive, chronic diseases. Carcinoma. Emaciation. Debility in morning. Marked regulating influence upon the glandular (sebaceous) secretions. Pre-senility. Ascites, in liver disease. Lycop. patient is thin, withered, full of gas and dry. Lacks vital heat; has poor circulation, cold extremities. Pains come and go suddenly. Sensitive to noise and odors.

Mind: Melancholy; afraid to be alone. Little things annoy, Extremely sensitive. Averse to undertaking new things. Head strong and haughty when sick. Loss of self-confidence. Hurried when eating. Constant fear of breaking down under stress. Apprehensive. Weak memory, confused thoughts; spells or writes wrong words and syllables. Failing brain-power (Anac; Phos; Baryt). Cannot bear to see anything new. Cannot read what he writes. Sadness in morning on awaking.

Head: Shakes head without apparent cause. Twists face and mouth. Pressing headache on vertex; worse from 4 to 8 pm, and from lying down or stooping, if not eating regularly (Cact). Throbbing headache after every paroxysm of coughing. Headaches over eyes in severe colds; better, uncovering (Sulph). Vertigo in morning on rising. Pain in temples, as if they were screwed toward each other. Tearing pain in occiput; better, fresh air. Great falling out of hair. Eczema; moist oozing behind ears. Deep furrows on forehead. Premature baldness and gray hair.

Eyes: Styes on lids near internal canthus. Day-blindness (Bothrops). Night-blindness more characteristic. Sees only one-half of an object. Ulceration and redness of lids. Eyes half open during sleep.

Ears: Thick, yellow, offensive discharge. Eczema about and behind ears. Otorrhœa and deafness with or without tinnitus; after scarlatina. Humming and roaring with hardness of hearing; every noise causes peculiar echo in ear.

Nose: Sense of smell very acute. Feeling of dryness posteriorly. Scanty excoriating, discharge anteriorly. Ulcerated nostrils. Crusts and elastic plugs (Kal b; Teuc). Fluent coryza. Nose stopped up. Snuffles; child starts from sleep rubbing nose. Fan-like motion of alae nasi (Kali brom; Phos).

Face: Grayish-yellow color of face, with blue circles around eyes. Withered, shriveled, and emaciated; copper-colored eruption. Dropping of lower jaw, in typhoid fever (Lach; Opium). Itching; scaly herpes in face and corner of mouth.

Mouth: Teeth excessively painful to touch. Toothache, with swelling of cheeks; relieved by warm application. Dryness of mouth and tongue, without thirst. Tongue dry, black, cracked, swollen; oscillates to and fro. Mouth waters. Blisters on tongue. Bad odor from mouth.

Throat: Dryness of throat, without thirst. Food and drink regurgitates through nose. Inflammation of throat, with stitches on swallowing; better, warm drinks. Swelling and suppuration of tonsils. Ulceration of tonsils, beginning on right side. Diphtheria; deposits spread from right to left; worse, cold drinks. Ulceration of vocal bands. Tubercular laryngitis, especially when ulceration commences.

Stomach: Dyspepsia due to farinaceous and fermentable food, cabbage, beans, etc. Excessive hunger. Aversion to bread, etc. Desire for sweet things. Food tastes sour. Sour eructations. Great weakness of digestion. Bulimia, with much bloating. After eating, pressure in stomach, with bitter taste in mouth. Eating ever so little creates fullness. Cannot eat oysters. Rolling of flatulence (Chin; Carb). Wakes at night feeling hungry. Hiccough. Incomplete burning eructations rise only to pharynx there burn for hours. Likes to take food and drink hot. Sinking sensation; worse night.

Abdomen: Immediately after a light meal, abdomen is bloated, full. Constant sense of fermentation in abdomen, like yeast working; upper left side. Hernia, right side. Liver sensitive. Brown spots on abdomen. Dropsy, due to hepatic disease. Hepatitis, atrophic form of nutmeg liver. Pain shooting across lower abdomen from right to left.

Stool: Diarrhoea. Inactive intestinal canal. Ineffectual urging. Stool hard, difficult, small, incomplete. Haemorrhoids; very painful to touch, aching (Mur ac).

Urine:	Pain in back before urinating; ceases after flow; slow in coming, must strain. Retention. Polyuria during the night. Heavy red sediment. Child cries before urinating (Bor).
Male:	No erectile power; impotence. Premature emission (Calad; Sel; Agn). Enlarge prostate. Condylomata.
Female:	Menses too late; last too long, too profuse. Vagina dry. Coition painful. Right ovarian pain. Varicose veins of pudenda. Leucorrhoea, acrid, with burning in vagina. Discharge of blood from genitals during stool.
Respiratory:	Tickling cough. Dyspnoea. Tensive, constrictive, burning pain in chest. Cough worse going down hill. Cough deep, hollow. Expectorations gray, thick, bloody, purulent, salty (Ars; Phos; Puls). Night cough, tickling as from Sulphur fumes. Catarrh of the chest in infants, seems full of mucus rattling. Neglected pneumonia, with great dyspnoea, flaying of alae nasae and presence of mucous rales.
Heart:	Aneurism (Baryta carb). Aortic disease. Palpitation at night. Cannot lie on left side.
Back:	Burning between scapulae as of hot coals. Pain in small of back.
Extremities:	Numbness, also drawing and tearing in limbs, especially while at rest or at night. Heaviness of arms. Tearing in shoulder and elbow joints. One foot hot, the other cold. Chronic gout, with chalky deposits in joints. Profuse sweat of the feet. Pain in heel on treading as from a pebble. Painful callosities on soles; toes and fingers contracted. Sciatica, worse right side. Cannot lie on painful side. Hands and feet numb. Right foot hot, left cold. Cramps in calves and toes at

night in bed. Limbs go to sleep. Twitching and jerking.

Fever: Chill between 3 and 4 pm, followed by sweat. Icy coldness. Feels as if lying on ice. One chill is followed by another (Calc; Sil; Hep).

Sleep: Drowsy during day. Starting in sleep. Dreams of accidents.

Skin: Ulcerates. Abscesses beneath skin; worse warm applications. Hives; worse, warmth. Violent itching; fissured eruptions. Acne. Chronic eczema associated with urinary, gastric and hepatic disorders; bleeds easily. Skin becomes thick and indurated. Varicose veins, naevi, erectile tumors. Brown spots, freckles worse on left side of face and nose. Dry, shrunken, especially palms; hair becomes prematurely gray. Dropsies. Offensive secretions; viscid and offensive perspiration, especially of feet and axilla. Psoriasis.

Modalities: Worse, right side, from right to left, from above downward, 4 to 8 pm; from heat or warm room, hot air, bed. Warm applications, except throat and stomach which are better from warm drinks. Better, by motion, after midnight, from warm food and drink, on getting cold, from being uncovered.

Relationship Complementary: Lycop acts with special benefit after Calcar and Sulphur. Iod; Graphites, Lach; Chelidon.

Antidotes: Camph; Puls; Caust.

Compare: Carbo-Nitrogenoid Constitution: Sulphur; Rhus; Urtica; Mercur; Hepar. Alumina (Lycop is the only vegetable that takes up aluminum. T. F. Allen) Ant c; Nat m; Ery; Nux; Bothrops (day-blindness; can scarcely see after sunrise; pain in right great toe). Plumbago littoralis-A Brazilian plant-- (Costive with red urine, pain in kidneys and joints and body generally; milky saliva, ulcerated mouth). Hydrast follows Lycop in indigestion.

Dose: Both the lower and the highest potencies are credited with excellent result. For purposes of aiding elimination the second and third attenuation of the Tincture, a few drops, 3 times a day, have proved efficacious, otherwise the 6th to 200th potency, and higher, in not too frequent doses.

A STUDY ON MATERIA MEDICA

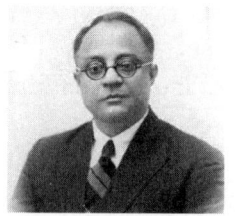

By: N.M. Choudhuri

N.M. Choudhuri was one of the eminent Indian homoeopaths. He was an alumnus of the Hering Medical College. He learned homoeopathy and was trained in Materia Medica by our old masters like Allen, Taylor and Farrington etc. He was principal and senior professor of Materia Medica at Bengal Allen Homoeopathic Medical College and Hospital Calcutta. He also served as editor of "Home & Homoeopathy" for a long time.

Being a disciple of the masters, mentioned, and teacher of the subject for a long time he had a deep insight into Materia Medica that emits its full light through his book "A Study on Materia Medica". Being a Materia Medica man he greatly emphasizes on the importance and accuracy in the study of the subject. He says in his lecture on Secale,

"A mistake in prescribing in such a case means to push our patient towards his or her grave. In our capacity as physicians and healers we possess unbounded opportunity to minister to people's wants and sufferings, but we must not forget, at the same time, that in us lies the power of doing an immense amount of harm to our fellow beings. The moment we relax in our effort to master the situation, we fall short of our duty and become guilty of unnecessary suffering to human beings. It behooves us, therefore, to be constantly on the alert and master every secret that our Materia Medica offers".

(N.M. Choudhuri, A Study on Materia Medica, P. 921)

A Study on Materia Medica" by N.M. Choudhuri is considered one of the important and useful books. Such a concise and clear way of teaching Materia Medica is rarely found in our literature. He has collected important features of some of very basic books in this volume. At the start of every remedy we read its keynote symptoms. This part can be a substitute of keynote books albeit the author has arranged these keynotes more briefly than Allen's and Lippe's. Then the author describes source of the remedy and elaborates its salient features in a very beautiful and lucid way. While describing an important feature of a remedy he compares it to analogous remedies; some time he contents only a list of comparable remedies as we see at bottom of remedies in Boericke's and some times he throws light on their characteristic and differentiating symptoms like Farrington. Differentiating remedies from one another is a difficul task in the study of Materia Medica and N.M. Choudhuri has emphatically worked out the same. He says in the preface,

"The principle of differentiation and assimilation then inculcated in me by these expounders has been given the greatest importance in this work. I will consider myself satisfied and my duty fulfilled, if I in my turn can impress on students and practitioners on this side of the hemisphere the essential importance of this most pivotal principle of this true science of the healing art."

(N.M. Choudhuri, A Study on Materia Medica, Preface)

Now we highlight the most important and a very useful feature of this book for which it excels many other books on the subject. Nearly at the end of every important remedy the author has incorporated some cases of eminent homoeopaths cured by it. This effectively makes the reader understand Materia Medica in a very practical way. Of course, N.M. Choudhuri was a successful teacher of Materia Medica and his book is concise, comprehensive, effective and practical.

It covers 441 remedies including all polychrests and many small/rare remedies like Cainca, Hoang Nan, Homarus, Slag and Sol etc. Let us, now, read a remedy from "A Study on Materia Medica",

ALOE SOCOTRINA
Keynotes

- An anti-psoric remedy.
- Weakness and loss of power of sphincter ani; insecurity of rectum.
- Great portal congestion, as seen in hemorrhoids and feeling of fullness and weight in the pelvis
- Moist, hot, itchy hemorrhoids protrude like a bunch of grapes, relieved by washing with cold water
- Loud rumbling and gurgling in the abdomen.
- Aggravation of symptoms after meals.

To write a materia medica without Aloe is to write a novel without a hero. Its importance and usefulness become evident as soon as we launch in our business of curing the sick. Its chief and the most important action is seen in the large intestines. Taken in a big dose it increases the intestinal secretion and its peristaltic action. It also produces sensation of heat, fullness, heaviness and throbbing in the rectum. In the homoeopathic therapeutics, Aloe justly assumes an important place in the treatment of diarrhea. I would like to give it in the very first place in those peculiar cases where the Aloe characteristics are present. As homoeopaths we have got no surer guide and no simpler process than to be guided by those characteristics. They are:

Firstly, a great feeling of weakness and loss of sphincter ani. This leads to a sensation of insecurity in the rectum. They afraid to pass flatus for fear stool will escape. In this Aloe resembles Oleander, Phosphorus, China, Hyoscyamus, Opium and Acidum phos. The urging for stool is great; he runs for the bathroom, but unfortunately even before he gets to it, his clothes are all soiled.

Secondly, a great feeling of fullness and weight in the pelvis as though the rectum were full of fecal matter which would fall out if not for the extreme caution.

Thirdly, loud rumbling and gurgling in the abdomen as though water were running out of bottle. This symptom when present in dysentery becomes a great characteristic.

Fourthly, the aggravation of the condition after eating each meal as in Arsenicum, China, Lycopodium, Podophyllum, Trombidium, Croton tig. and Ferrum.

Aloe causes great portal congestions and as is usually the case in all such remedies we notice a great depression, lassitude and languor clouding their mental atmosphere. They are fleshy and phlegmatic, highly dissatisfied and angry about themselves. They consider life as almost a burden and carry on their existence in a sad, dispirited sort of way. They are inclined to suffer from congestion of the head and hence a dull frontal headache with heaviness of the eyes is common. Sometimes the headache alternate with lumbago. They suffer from pain deep in the orbits and have yellow vision. The congestion of the portal system referred to above gives them a sensation of constant fullness and heaviness in the abdomen. Rumbling in the abdomen, constant discharge of flatus, a feeling of weakness in the abdomen, as if diarrhea would set in, great cutting, griping pain in the right and lower portion of abdomen, a sensation of plug between symphisis pubis and os coccyx, urging to stool, constant bearing down in rectum are symptoms that ought to be remembered. The character of the Aloe stool also is equally striking. It is mostly transparent, jelly like in dysentery and yellow semi-liquid fecal in diarrhea. This diarrhea is always worse while walking or standing and is often followed by great prostration and fainting spells.

The hemorrhoids of Aloe, the result of the same portal congestions, protrude like a bunch of grapes. Constant backache, the same bearing down sensation in the rectum, the sensation of fullness described above should be our important landmarks in the selection of the remedy. The hemorrhoids are mostly moist due to constant mucus secretion from the anus. They are very tender, sore, hot, itchy and are generally relieved by washing it with cold water.

In this connection we may think of Bromium, and Muriaticum acidum, two remedies equally great in hemorrhoids. It differs from the former in the fact that Bromium piles are relieved by application of saliva and from Muriaticum acidum by its relief from application of warm water.

The constipation of Aloe is equally prominent because of the same want of confidence in the sphincter ani. I remember quite vividly a case of a little boy about five years old that was brought to our clinic years ago, when I was a student in the Hering Medical College of Chicago. He used to soil his clothes at all odd times with hard lumpy stools, which his mother ascribed to sheer wickedness on his part. When cane failed and the trouble grew worse, he was brought to the clinic. A few doses of Aloe put and end to all his unintentional villany.

Aloe is a deeply anti-psoric remedy and it is of special use in chronic cases when the above symptoms are well marked.

Case 1

A German woman, aged seventy two, had been a hard worker; married nearly fifty years, and reared a large family of children. Complained of severe pain in abdomen. Her husband called, and not being able to talk english, the doctor derived but little information. Gave Nux-v. and Dios., to be given alternately. Two weeks later patient's daughter called, reporting her mother no better. Doctor called to see her, found pulse 100, full, skin hot and dry; tongue, covered with heavy white fur and quite dry; lips dry and sore; much thirst, desire for cold and sour. Had been a habitual cider drinker. Anything cold aggravated the complaint, causing more frequent passages and pain. Stools were very frequent, especially from 4 to 10 a.m. consisting of stringy mucus of yellow color, and occasionally mixed with foul material. Desire for stool come on suddenly; could hardly get off her bed quick enough before some of the stool would escape. Any attempt to pass urine, would be accompanied with flow of stool. Stools accompanied with much flatulence, and were preceded with much pain in hypogastrium and sacrum, which relieved by passage of stool. Symptoms all worse in forenoon. Patient was irritable and angry because she was sick. Aloe 20 trituration, every two hours. Two days later, found patient worse, very much prostrated and fever still present. First dose of Aloe was followed with intense headache, tearing and pressing in character, confined to the left side of head and worse in fore part of the day; relieved somewhat by tying a handkerchief tightly about the head. Regarding this as aggravation of the remedy, two doses were ordered to be given daily of the same remedy. Three days latter, the patient was found to be much better in every respect.

Dr. G. J. Jones

Case 2

Mr. C. H. B., aged fifty five, gentleman, July13. Has been troubled excessively for six years with what he termed "moist piles" for which he had in vain tried allopathic and homoeopathic treatment, here and in Europe. He complained of his linen being constantly stained by mucus discharge from the anus; bowels generally moved once a day; stool covered with slime; after stool, feels "played out"; is always worse after bating; at times, the discharge is so disagreeable and annoying that he feels like shooting himself. Prescribed Ant-c 1M which was repeated in August, and again on October 17, when he wrote me: "The whole thing has experienced a great change for the better since taking your few powders; for while, formerly, the spongy substance was most always passing off, here is only now and then some of this mucus whitish stuff, which is wiped off." Very little if any, improvement followed until January 3, 1875, when I prescribed Aloe 30, to be taken in water a teaspoonful, night and morning for one week, the indication being "gob-like evacuation of clear jelly, with faintness for hours afterwards, and anxiousness on account of health; a kind of chill running through the system, with pressure on the bladder, chill disappearing at once after making water." Aloe relieved markedly until February 4, when the prescription was repeated. May 27, my patient came again, after having been troubled for six weeks, and this time he gave me another indication of Aloe, viz., " always much worse during hot, damp weather." Aloe, one dose every day, was followed by rapid improvement and now (August 3) my patient considers himself radically cured.

Dr. C. Mohr, Jr

MATERIA MEDICA OF HOMOEOPATHIC MEDICINES

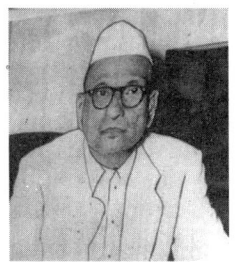

By S.R. Phatak

S.R. Phatak is an eminent Indian homoeopath. He authored the following useful books.

1. Materia Medica of Homoeopathic Medicines
2. A Concise Repertory of Homoeopathic Medicines
3. Repertory of Biochemic Remedies
4. Repertory of Homoeopathic Medicines (Marathi)

Phatak's Materia Medica of Homoeopathic Medicines bears a number of useful features for which it becomes a living Materia Medica. Some of its virtues are as follows,

We know that our short Materia Medica books, like Boericke's, Boger's etc. do not contain complete symptoms of a given remedy. Every author provides or emphasizes some of important characteristic and common symptoms according to his personal experience and choice. One has to go through many Materia Medicas in order to know all the important and characteristic symptoms of a remedy. Phatak tries to solve this problem and provides a rich collection of characteristic symptoms taken from different books.

He says in his preface,

"In compiling this Materia Medica, I have included all the symptoms given by Boger. I have tried to simplify many of his ambiguous words by explaining their meaning. Moreover, I have garnered many useful clinical and other symptoms from other Materia Medicas (which were not given by Boger) and have included them here".

The second beautiful feature is its easy comprehensive language and text. Our old books written two or one century ago contain many words and terms not in use now. A modern student feels extremely hard to understand such old terminology. While collecting and presenting symptoms from Boger's "Synoptic Key" and other Materia Medicas Phatak explains such ambiguities and makes them easy and comprehensible. Difficult words used even by Phatak have been replaced by easy words in the B.Jain's second edition. This is highlighted in the preface to the second edition,

"Words or clinical terminology that are rarely used and are not likely to be understood easily have been replaced by contemporary language".

This makes Phatak's Materia Medica a handy and friendly book for the modern homoeopathic students.

Phatak, like Boericke, interlinks symptoms of a remedy to different pathological conditions of particular names. It also has a unique index of drugs useful to surgeons. These features make this book a practical Materia Medica for those who come from conventional medicine into homoeopathy. Gunavante says,

"Though not containing as many remedies as Boericke's, this book covers a wider spectrum of each remedy, especially the mental aspect, thus qualifying it as essential for reference before any other Materia Medica".

(Gunavante, Introduction to Homoeopathic Prescribing, P. 42)

It covers 415 remedies including nearly all polychrests and many rares. Three types of letters (block, italic and roman) have been used to show the relative value of symptoms. Publisher's note at back of the second edition,

"A brief materia medica derived primarily from the work of Boger, with additions. While most practitioners in the

USA, who wanted a small "Pocket Manual", often chose the Boericke's work, many in the UK preferred Phatak's work. In a comparison between them one may find Phatak to be a bit more readable. Those who have used it say that the summaries he presents of the remedies contain useful details that are not found in Boericke's".

CHINA OFFICINALIS

Generalities: This was the first remedy proved by Dr. Hahnemann. It affects the blood, making it thinner, and impoverished. It weakens the heart and impairs the CIRCULATION, producing congestion and HEMORRHAGE, anemia, complete relaxation and collapse. The debility in China, is due to PROFUSE EXHAUSTING DISCHARGES, loss of vital fluid, excessive suppuration, diarrhea, hemorrhages, etc. INTERMITTENT, periodicity is very marked in fever and neuralgia. Patient becomes weak, oversensitive and nervous; everything upsets him---light, noise, odor, pain, etc. Bursting pain. Neuralgia. Dropsy after loss of fluid, hemorrhage. Emaciation esp. of children. Anaemia. Hard swelling. Rheumatism. Sepsis. Inflammation of bleeding organ, after hemorrhages, and the part rapidly becomes black. Convulsion during hemorrhage. Hemorrhage, profuse, with loss of sight, faintness, and ringing in ears. Post-operative gas pain not > from passing it. Ill effect of masturbation, vexation, cold, stopped coryza, tea, mercury, alcohol. Psoas abscess. It is suited to persons of thin, dry, bilious constitutions. Wounds become black and gangrenous. Epilepsy; chorea; paralysis; from loss of fluids.

Worse: VITAL LOSS. TOUCH. Jar. Noise. PERIODICITY; alternate days. Cold winds, drafts. Open air. Eating. Fruits. Milk. Impure water. Spoiled fish, meat. Tea. Mental exertion. During and after stool. Smoking. Autumn, summer.

Better: Hard pressure. Loose clothes. Bending double. In room; warmth.

Mind: Disobedient, stubborn, contempt for everything. Fixed idea, that he is unhappy, persecuted by enemies. Disposition to hurt other people's feelings. Fear of dogs and other animals, at night. Sudden crying and tossing about, when cheerful. Ill-humor, < petting and caressing. Dislike for all mental and physical work. Builds air castles. Indifference, sad, no desire to live. Wants to commit suicide but lacks courage. Reluctant to speak. Mistakes in speech and writing. Spoonerism. Loss of control over mind.

Head: Bursting, throbbing pain, with throbbing of carotids. Sensation as if brain were swashing to and fro., causing pain; bruised pain in brain,< temples. Vertigo, falls backward while walking. Stitches from temple to temple. Sore sensitive scalp, < touching or combing hair. Headache, < in the sun, > by moving head up and down, hard pressure, rubbing. Sweats when walking in open air. Head heavy.

Eyes: Blue color around eyes. Night blindness, due to anemic retina. Scalding tears. Pressure in eyes as from drowsiness. Black spots before eyes. Pupils dilated. Intermittent ciliary neuralgia. Smart as from salt. Stitching as from sand. Eyes painful on reading and writing.

Ears: Red, hot. Ringing in ears, with headache. Tinnitus then vertigo. Stitches in ears. Hardness

Nose:	of hearing. Foul, purulent, bloody discharge. Ill-effects of suppressed coryza---headache. Habitual easy bleeding from nose, esp. morning on rising. Smell too acute. Cold sweat about nose. Nose hot, red. Violent dry sneezing.
Face:	Earthy, sickly, pale; Hippocratic, bluish around the eyes. Face bloated; red. Lips dry, blackish and shriveled swelling of veins. Red hot face, with cold hands. Flushed after hemorrhage, sexual excess, loss of vital fluid, in coma.
Mouth:	Toothache while infant sucks the breast, > by pressing teeth firmly together and by warmth. Toothache with sweat. Food tastes bitter, even water, or too salty. Thongue; thick, dry-coated; tip burns, followed by salivation. Taste bitter, salty or acute. Gums swollen.
Stomach:	Bitter or sour eructations, after milk. Craving; for dainty; sour or sweet things, highly seasoned food, desires various things without knowing what (children). Quick satiety. Anorexia, feels satiated all the time, aversion, to all food, to bread, butter, coffee. Voracious appetite in emaciation of children. Loud belching without relief. Digestion slow. Milk disagrees. Weight, after eating small quantity of food. Ill effects of tea. Cold feeling in stomach. Thirst for cold water that < diarrhoea. Pulsations and rumbling, in epigastrium. Frequent vomiting. Hichough. Hematemasis. Stomach sore. Fermetation after eating fruits. Thirst during apyrexia; before chill. Hungry and yet want of appetie; only while eating some appetite and natural taste for food return.
Abdomen:	Liver and spleen enlarged. Flatulent bloating; >motion. Colic> by bending double. Post operative gas pains, no relief from passing

it. Heat in abdomen as if hot water running down. Periodical liver symptoms. Pain from rectum to genitals. Gall stone colic. Jaundice; after leucorrhea, masturbation, sexual excess, diarrhoea. Stools; lienteric; dark, foul; watery; Bloody; painless; < eating; at night, from fruits; milk, beer, during hot weather. Diarrhoea; after weaning, in children; chronic in children, who become drowsy, pupils dilated, body becomes cold esp. chin, nose and rapid respiration. Involuntary stools.

Urinary: Frequent urination. Burning at meatus <rubbing of clothes. Urine turbid, dark, scanty. Pinkish sediment. Hematuria. Enuresis of weakly children.

Male: Impotence, or morbid sexual desire, with lascivious fancies. Frequent emissions followed by great weakness. Swelling testes and spermatic cord --- after gonorrhoea. Orchitis. Sexual desire, with craving for dainties.

Female: Ovaritis from sexual excess. Desire too strong in lying-in women. Menses; too early, dark, profuse, clotted, with abdominal distention. Bloody leukorrhea; seems to take blood dark, with fainting, convulsions. Asphyxia of new born due to great loss of blood by the mother. Painful induration in the vagina.

Respiration: Hemoptisis. Puffy, rattling breathing, suffocative catarrh; connot breathe with head low. Asthma; < damp weather, autumn or after depletion. Every motion excites palpitation and takes his breath. Painfully sore chest with a soreness between scapulae, cannot bear percussion or auscultation. Suppurative phthisis. Paroxysms of cough after eating or laughing < evening,

	night. Wants to be fanned but not too hard for it takes her breath.
Heart:	Every movement excites palpitation.
Neck & Back:	Pressure as of a stone between scapulae. Interscapular spine painful. Sharp pains across kidneys < movement, at night. Knife like pains around the back. Heavy pressure on sacrum. Backache as from sitting bent for long time. Lumbago < slight motion.
Extremeities:	As if heavy load on shoulders. Spasmodic stretching of arms, with clenched fingers. Hands trembles (while writing). Twitching in knees. Sensation as of a band around legs, or arms. One hand is icy cold other is warm. Swelling of veins of the hands. Nails blue. Pain in libms and joints feel as if sprained < slight touch; > hard pressure. Weariness of joints < morning, sitting. Pain in marrow. Caries of bones with profuse sweat.
Skin:	Extreme sensitiveness to touch; hard pressure relieves. Dermatitis. Humid gangrene. Yellow color.
Sleep:	Drowsiness. Heavy, snoring sleep; esp. in children. Anxious frightful dreams; fear of dream remains. Sleeplessness as a prodrome.
Fever:	Marked prodrome. Stages of chill, heat and sweat well marked. Chill, then thirst, then heat, then thirst. Chill begins in the breast. Red hot face, with cold hands. Hectic fever. DRENCHING SWEATS; AT NIGHT; < least motion; from weakness; from depletions etc. Tropical fevers. Sepsis.

COMPLEMENTARY: Carb-v., Ferr., Kali-c.

RELATED: Carb-v.

Bibliography

1. Allen, H C, *Key Notes (4th Edition)*, Homoeopathic Stores & Hospital, Lahore, Pakistan.
2. Banerjea, S K 1999, *Miasmatic Diagnosis*, B.Jain Publishers, New Delhi, India.
3. Boericke, Garth 1976, *Principles of Homoeopathy*, Homoeopathic Stores & Hospital, Lahore, Pakistan.
4. Boericke W, *Pocket Manual of Homoeopathic Materia Medica*, Twelfth edition. n.d., Homoeopathic Stores & Hospital, Lahore, Pakistan.
5. Boger, C M 1999. *The Study of Materia Medica and Taking the Case*, B.Jain Publishers, New Delhi, India.
6. Choudhery, Ahmad Hassan 1994, *Homoeopathic Repertory ka Istemal* (Urdu), Homeopathic Research Centre, Sargodha.
7. Choudhury, Harimohan 1986, *50 Millesimal Potency in Theory and Practice*, B.Jain Publishers, New Delhi, India.
8. Choudhury, N M 2009, *A Study on Materia Medica*, B.Jain Publishers, New Delhi, India.
9. Close, Stuart 1999, *The Genius of Homoeopathy*, B.Jain Publishers, New Delhi, India.
10. Farrington, E A 2002, *Lectures on Clinical Materia Medica in Family Order* B.Jain Publishers, New Delhi, India.
11. Gaskin, A 1995, *Comparative Study on Kent's Materia Medica*, B.Jain Publishers, New Delhi, India.
12. Gunavante 1998, *Introduction to Homoeopathic Prescribing*, B.Jain Publishers, New Delhi, India.
13. Gunavante, S M, *Genius of Homoeopathic Remedies*, B.Jain Publishers, New Delhi, India.
14. Hahnemann, Samuel 1997, *Organon of Medicine* B.Jain Publishers, New Delhi, India.
15. Hahnemann, Samuel 1986, *Organon of Medicine "Dudgeon's Translation"*, B.Jain Publishers, New Delhi, India.

16. Kent, J T 1999, *Lectures on Homeopathic Philosophy*, B.Jain Publishers, New Delhi, India.
17. Kent, J T 1999 *Lectures on Homeopathic Materia Medica*, B.Jain Publishers, New Delhi, India.
18. Kent, J T, *Repertory of the Homoeopathic Materia Medica*, 2nd Edition, Masood Publications, Lahore, Pakistan.
19. Kent, J T 1992, *Lesser Writings*, B.Jain Publishers, New Delhi, India.
20. Kishore, Jugal 1999, *Kent's Lectures on Materia Medica* [Introduction] B.Jain Publishers, New Delhi, India.
21. Lippe, A V, *Key Notes and Red Line Symptoms of the Materia Medica*, Indian Books & Periodicals Syndicate (n.d.), New Delhi, India.
22. Nash, E.B, *Leaders in Homoeopathic Therapeutics*, (7th Edition) Homoeopathic Stores & Hospital, Lahore, Pakistan.
23. Phatak, S R 1999, *Materia Medica of Homoeopathic Medicines*, B.Jain Publishers, New Delhi, India.
24. Roberts, H A 1992, *Principles and Art of Cure by Homoeopathy* B.Jain Publishers, New Delhi, India.
25. Herbert A Roberts, *Sensation As If*, Homoeopathic Stores & Hospital, Lahore, Pakistan.
26. Sankaran, P 1976, *The Study of Materia Medica*, The Homoeopathic Medical Publications, Bombay, India.
27. Schmidt, Pierre, *The Art of Case Taking*, B.Jain Publishers, New Delhi, India.
28. Tyler, M L, *Homoeopathic Drug Picture*, Medical Book Center, Lahore, Pakistan.
29. Tyler, M L & Weir, John, *Repertorizing* (Printed in *Kent's Repertory of the Homoeopathic Materia Medica*) (2nd Edition) Masood Publications, Lahore, Pakistan.
30. Vithoulkas, George 1998, *The Science of Homoeopathy*, B.Jain Publishers, New Delhi, India.
31. Yasgur, Jay 2003, *Homoeopathic Dictionary*, B.Jain Publishers, New Delhi, India.

REVIEWS

Whom should I congratulate Dr. Mir or Dr. Kathy Desjardins or the fertile intercourse between the two should be appreciated that helped conceiving and making this beautiful book? My praise and appreciation for all!

Now a few words for this book. While homoeopathic materia medica is our main armamentarium that is used in the fight against disease and ill health, a fuller knowledge of its components, designs and purposes is presented nowhere in lucid and compact form for the students of homoeopathy. This was Dr. Mir's share that he felt this need of the beginners and met the same for them successfully. Dr. Mir's book is a practical guide to the study and use of homoeopathic materia medica and it demonstrates successfully the use and importance of different types of symptoms, sensations, modalities, causations and conditions that comprise the portraits and individualities of our medicines. Thus by making the study of materia medica a living, dynamic and enjoyable process, Dr. Mir has contributed a valuable treatise to the literature of homoeopathy.

Now my advice to the student---Read Dr. Mir's book, start your study of Nash, Kent and George, assimilate the law of cure and enjoy serenity and tranquility by performing valuable cures.

Dr. Chaudhery Ahmad Hassan.
19 September 2008.
Sargodha, Pakistan.

In the last few decades, more than 2000 new remedy names have appeared in homeopathic literature. There have been many philosophical advancements too, leading to varied interpretation and use of our Materia Medica. Many new books covering new remedies, consolidating historical data and text books for students have been published. But there have been few attempts to present the study of Materia Medica in a systematic and coherent way. Dr. Zahed's book "UNDERSTANDING & UTILIZING The Homoeopathic Materia Medica" fills this gap. This work covers different facets of our remedies, discusses relative merit of different symptoms, different approaches to study them, explores the existing literature and presents the data in a very lucid manner. Students, who often get confused due to the mass of information in our medicines, will find this book very useful. I hope this work will serve as a guide to our young students for many years to come and illuminate the path for studying our Materia Medica.

Warm wishes,

Dr. Manish Bhatia

Dr. Manish Bhatia
22nd May 2008
Jaipur

The practice of homeopathy in the 21st century is both a skilled art and a complex science. Consequently, it is a difficult discipline to master. Successful homeopaths know this and devote time exploring ways in which they can perfect their art in order to best serve their patients. As James Compton-Burnett wrote: The fact is we need any and every way of finding the right remedy.

Being well-versed in classical theories is as important as getting to grips with contemporary methodologies and this is where Dr Zahed's book is useful. For the beginner homeopathic student, this book provides invaluable insight into the use of one of our tools of trade – the materia medica. The first chapter title hints at the content of the book – to memorize or to understand! Dr Zahed knows that in order to master materia medica, we must first understand it. Rote learning will only allow us to pass tests. So, it is only through understanding that practitioners will be able to utilize the treasures held within the materia medica.

And this is what Dr Zahed's book does. It takes us on a journey of discovery in which the characteristics of materia medica and the terminology associated with it are explained clearly and with vigour.

A useful chapter on potency presents the reader with a wide range of traditional viewpoints. This is a difficult subject. However, Dr Zahed's summary at the end of the chapter adds clarity.

Liberal use of quotes from the homeopathic masters, as well as case examples, add interest to the text.

This is a useful book for a student of homeopathy which facilitates understanding of some basic principles. Hopefully it will also stimulate interest in further research of masters' work and perhaps even arouse curiosity about contemporary homeopathy.

Congratulations to Dr. Zahed for simplifying the study of materia medica and making it accessible to newcomers.

Kathy Thomas
RCHom, Advanced Diploma in Homeopathy (NZ)
Senior Lecturer and Associate Principal of Homeopathy
(South Pacific College of Homeopathy)

Knowledge, in all its aspects, brings our understanding to the fore and for excellence in prescribing knowledge is always an essential ingredient. Who we are as a person is the most important factor in how we live our life, and thus also in how we practice as a homoeopath. Dr. Zahed's 'Understanding & Utilizing The Homoeopathic Materia Medica', a superb collection of his essays & lectures, weaves these insights, among many others, into the fabric of what homeopathy is, how it works and what it means to be a homeopath.

The author has spared himself no pains in his endeavour to present the main ideas in the simplest and most intelligible form, and on the whole, in the sequence and connection in which they actually originated. The wealth of detail, the infinite care never to let anything pass unexplained, with which he presented to the students of Homoeopathy the result of his experience, are impressive & worth appreciating. All in this entire book is not only to be recommended to homoeopaths, but I would say it is a "must". But not only a must, it's a delight and a joy to have it and work with it.

With Warm Wishes,
Dr. Navneet Bidani
Director Dr. Bidani's
Centre for Homoeopathy.
www.drbidani.co.nr

Dear Dr. Mir

First of all, let me congratulate you on the wonderful piece of love that you have produced. It leaves me with no doubt in my mind that it will go a long way in helping beginners as well the experienced professionals understand the intricacies of our huge MM and understanding the remedy picture a lot better.

Please find my comments in red. All places where I have placed a word in bracket, it is essentially a semantic suggestion where I felt a different word or expression could be used. In other place I have put my comments.

You will find that most of my observations stem from a difference in philosophy. I have always had differences with the Kentian mode of Repertorization and based my treatment on the method suggested by Hahnemann and Boenningheusen. For me the disease picture consists of the following:

1. Aetiology/Causation
2. Symptom Complex
   - Locations
   - Sensations
   - Modalities
3. Concomitant Symptoms
4. Miasms

In addition, the only symptoms important to me are the current diseased state that represents the deviation from the earlier state of health.

Hence, my suggestions are not necessarily meant to be incorporated. They are more pertaining to a different school of thought.

Once again, accept my congratulatory note for this beautiful book.

With Warm regards,
Niel Madhavan